MEN IN THERAPY
The Challenge of Change

THE GUILFORD FAMILY THERAPY SERIES
Alan S. Gurman, *Editor*

Recent volumes

MEN IN THERAPY: THE CHALLENGE OF CHANGE
Richard L. Meth and Robert S. Pasick with Barry Gordon,
Jo Ann Allen, Larry B. Feldman, and Sylvia Gordon

FAMILY SYSTEMS IN MEDICINE
Christian N. Ramsey, Jr., *Editor*

NEGOTIATING PARENT-ADOLESCENT CONFLICT:
A BEHAVIORAL-FAMILY SYSTEMS APPROACH
Arthur L. Robin and Sharon L. Foster

FAMILY TRANSITIONS: CONTINUITY AND CHANGE
OVER THE LIFE CYCLE
Celia Jaes Falicov, *Editor*

FAMILIES AND LARGER SYSTEMS: A FAMILY THERAPIST'S GUIDE
THROUGH THE LABYRINTH
Evan Imber-Black

AFFECTIVE DISORDERS AND THE FAMILY:
ASSESSMENT AND TREATMENT
John F. Clarkin, Gretchen Haas, and Ira D. Glick, *Editors*

HANDBOOK OF FAMILY THERAPY TRAINING
AND SUPERVISION
Howard A. Liddle, Douglas C. Breunlin, and Richard C. Schwartz, *Editors*

MARITAL THERAPY: AN INTEGRATIVE APPROACH
William C. Nichols

FAMILY THERAPY SOURCEBOOK
Fred P. Piercy, Douglas H. Sprenkle, and Associates

SYSTEMIC FAMILY THERAPY: AN INTEGRATIVE APPROACH
William C. Nichols and Craig A. Everett

MEN IN THERAPY
The Challenge of Change

RICHARD L. METH and ROBERT S. PASICK

with

Barry Gordon, Jo Ann Allen
Larry B. Feldman, Sylvia Gordon

THE GUILFORD PRESS
New York   London

© 1990 The Guilford Press
A Division of Guilford Publications, Inc.
72 Spring Street, New York, NY 10012

Printed in the United States of America

This book is printed on acid-free paper.

Last digit is print number: 9 8 7 6 5 4

Library of Congress Cataloging-in-Publication Data

Meth, Richard L.
    Men in therapy : the challenge of change / Richard L. Meth and
Robert S. Pasick with Barry Gordon . . . [et al.].
        p.   cm. — (Guilford family therapy series)
    Includes bibliographical references.
    ISBN 0-89862-104-6   ISBN 0-89862-485-1 (pbk)
    1. Men—Mental health.   2. Psychotherapy.   3. Men—Psychology.
I. Pasick, Robert S.   II. Title.   III. Series.
RC451.4.M45M47   1990
616.89′0081—dc20   89-49684
                                                             CIP

Dedicated to our families:
past and present

Authors

Jo Ann Allen, M.S.W. Faculty member of the University of Michigan School of Social Work and practitioner of family therapy at the Ann Arbor Center for the Family.

Larry B. Feldman, M.D. Clinical Associate Professor, Department of Psychiatry, Loyola University of Chicago Medical School, Maywood, Illinois.

Barry Gordon, Ph.D. Clinical psychologist in private practice in Cleveland, Ohio.

Sylvia Gordon, Ph.D. Practitioner of family therapy at the Ann Arbor Center for the Family.

Richard L. Meth, M.S.W. Director, Center for Marital and Family Therapy, School of Family Studies, University of Connecticut, Storrs, Connecticut.

Robert S. Pasick, Ph.D. Psychologist, family therapist, and consultant at the Ann Arbor Center for the Family. Conducts workshops on Gender Issues in the Workplace.

Foreword

This is a book about men and about men in therapy. It is about the inner life of men, their relationships, their lives at work and in their families.

But aren't all books on psychological development, on adult life, on therapy about men? Carol Gilligan, among others, has pointed out that our vision of the human experience, of psychological and social function and dysfunction has been constructed primarily by and about men. Male ways of being and ways of knowing have been defined as the desirable norm while women have been defined as "other." But in another sense, although psychological writing has been androcentric, it has also been gender blind. It has assumed a male perspective but has not really explored what it means to be a man any more than what it means to be a woman.

The authors of this volume take a different path. They explore the roles and expectations of men in our society. They hold the outcomes of gender socialization and gender stereotyping up for examination and for criticism.

This volume could be described as expressing a feminist perspective on men. That, however, is not altogether accurate. It does draw from feminism the central importance of gender and of the deeply embedded gender stereotypes that circumscribe and limit the potential of men as well as women. It challenges these stereotypes and takes a position, reminiscent of feminist therapy, that one of the goals of treatment is to liberate men from the bondage of dysfunctional sex role prescriptions. The fact that there is no parallel word, no language which describes this lens when focused on the world of men perhaps indicates how unusual and innovative this perspective is. It is certainly not "masculine." The term "gender sensitive" is used but gender sensitive is too passive, it implies neither a critical nor proactive stance. These authors are sensitive to gender issues but they also critique and prescribe action, not only in therapy but in the world. They take the position that much of male socialization in our society has not been good for men, that it inhibits men's development and the full realization of their potential, particularly in relationships, as husbands, fathers, lovers, sons, and friends.

The volume not only critiques but prescribes a therapeutic focus and therapeutic interventions that can truly liberate men. It teaches us how to help men engage in the therapeutic process, a process in itself in conflict with male norms. It describes and illustrates through rich cases examples how to help men encounter and rework their identity as males through revisiting their relationships with their fathers. The central and crucial role of rigid gendered behaviors in marital conflict is explained and ways of liberating both men and women from oppressive images of marriage are presented. And ways of helping men help each other through the use of groups is demonstrated and the potential of men's friendships expanded. Such therapy can help individual men but also implicit in this stance is a call for major social change. Such change, however, as we have learned in the women's movement is a long time coming, particularly in the face of powerful social, political, and economic forces that support the continued dichotomization of the human world into stereotypical male and female images. Until our society and socialization processes are altered, this book can guide us as we help men overcome the limitations placed on them by gender stereotypes and become agents of change in their world.

ANN HARTMAN

Preface

This book addresses two central questions: (1) What are the effects of gender role conditioning on men's lives? and (2) How can therapists help men change so that their lives are less dominated by the dysfunctional effects of such conditioning? In many ways it is a beginning step, intended to serve as an opening statement about men's lives and the role of therapy in helping men change.

Unfortunately, relatively little effort has been devoted to the study of male gender role conditioning. This was manifest during a visit by one of the authors to a bookstore in search of research material about this subject. When the manager was asked if there was a section for books on men and masculinity, he looked puzzled and admitted that they did not have a specific section of such books. Then he smiled and swept his arm over the aisles and said, "Almost all of the books in this store are about men and masculinity."

In one sense the manager was right. A great many books have been devoted to accounts of men living out the stereotyped roles to which they have been socialized—for example, the strong fearless athlete venerated for playing through pain; the hard-working, hard-playing, hard-drinking factory worker; the successful, cocksure Wall Street businessman. However, very few books have examined the deleterious emotional and interpersonal consequences of masculine stereotyping. This book will closely examine these consequences and explore ways in which therapists can help men overcome them.

The tone of books written about men or by men in the past few years has often tended to be critical, chastising men for being emotional cave dwellers. This book attempts to go beyond such a negative focus, and tries to identify a basis for understanding male behavior which can be used to help change it. It also examines many of the forces that have shaped men and tended to limit them to their traditional roles and behaviors.

Understanding men requires us to recognize the variety of influences on them. Within the family each man's experience is determined by the interaction of many forces: temperament, parental relationships, sibling relationships, etc. These alone however do not shape and guide a man in his pursuit of manhood. Larger systems such as the workplace, the media, and public policy barrage men with powerful messages that tell men how to think and behave as men. Gender sensitive therapy requires that the clinician be vigilant to the impact of all of these systems.

The issue of gender has long been ignored by clinicians. Although we do not presume that every problem men bring to therapy is gender-related, we do believe that many of them are caused by the rigid societal prescriptions that dictate how men should and should not act, think, and feel. We hope that this book will increase the reader's awareness of gender conditioning as it relates to effective therapy.

Working with men in individual, marital, family, or group therapy necessarily requires a high degree of personal involvement. Regardless of the therapeutic approach, every clinician brings to his work attitudes toward and about men that have the potential to interfere with effective therapy. It is essential that clinicians be aware of these attitudes and use this awareness to enhance, rather than diminish, their ability to help men change.

While we believe that the issues discussed in this book are applicable to all men in American society, the specific examples we present necessarily focus on the group most often seen in our clinical practices—middle class, heterosexual men. In the clinical examples presented, the reader will meet men working as manual laborers and bank vice-presidents, self-employed small business owners and physicians. Some are single, some are married without children, some are fathers, some are divorced. All have been heavily influenced by gender role stereotyping and the myths that such stereotyping perpetuates.

The genesis of the book dates back to 1982, when Richard Meth and Robert Pasick met at an annual meeting of the American Family Therapy Association. At a special session described as a discussion on men's issues, twenty men voluntarily shared their perspectives on being men, raising children, and working with men in therapy. Through their conversation they were delighted to learn they were not alone in their feelings of isolation. From this initial encounter their friendship grew and developed each year at the annual AFTA meetings.

Once a year they returned to this group and discussed their lives and experiences as men and as therapists working with men. Aware of how few resources were available, they decided to write a book about men and therapy. At first, this was to be a two-way project. However, after a few months the immense scope of it began to be overwhelming. With schedules already bursting at the seams, it seemed that this task would require them to take extended leaves from their work and families to complete it—a process that seemed to mirror the male dilemma they had spent hours discussing. While each recognized how all consuming writing such a book could be, neither felt it "manly" to admit it. Afraid to let the other down, it took them a while to finally confess, with some relief, their mutual dilemma, and to agree that a change in format was needed.

They decided to solicit friends for help. Richard contacted Larry Feldman in Chicago, a colleague and founder of the men's interest group at AFTA. Robert recruited Barry Gordon from Cleveland, a graduate school friend, and Jo Ann Allen and Sylvia Gordon, with whom he was working on a gender project at the Ann Arbor Center for the Family.

By changing the format the six of us have been able to achieve a collaborative effort. We have met many times to formulate ideas we wanted to present and revised each other's work throughout the process. Several chapters have been co-authored. In many ways, the production of this book itself counters the typical "male" method of work, an approach where men work alone in a competitive spirit. Here, collaboration and cooperation have replaced autonomy and competition. Although Richard Meth and Robert Pasick were responsible for outlining the structure of the book, each author has made substantial contributions that we believe have produced a comprehensive analysis.

Our work is presented in two parts: Understanding Men in U.S. Society, and Men in the Process of Change. The first part shows men in various roles—workers, husbands, fathers and friends. Chapter 1 begins by exploring in general terms how males are conditioned to think about masculinity and what is expected of them as men in our society. We examine how many of these social constructs about being male restrict the growth and range of men's behavior. Chapter 2 is devoted to a detailed exploration of how men are raised to work. Chapter 3 looks at the psychosocial underpinnings of how men relate to women, particularly as spouses. Chapter 4 examines men as fathers. A common theme linking these chapters is the strong conditioning that men receive about the central importance of working and being "good providers" for their families. The last chapter in this part, Chapter 5, focuses on men's friendships with other men.

The second part, Men in the Process of Change, addresses how best to help men overcome common problems. It provides a treatment chapter for each topic examined in the first part. Our approach is an integration of several theoretical schools, including family systems, humanistic, experiential, psychoeducational, psychodynamic, and behavioral. Much of our therapy offers men information on the negative consequences of gender role stereotypes as a way of helping them enact meaningful change. Clinical vignettes and examples from the media are frequently utilized to punctuate the ways in which clinicians can intervene.

We are at an important juncture in relating between the genders. The changes that have occurred for women as a result of the feminist movement have left men confused and uncertain. Internalized images that have served as guides for many men no longer apply. Men need help working on the changes that they can commit to for their own development and to improve their relationships with women, children, and other men. Many men are beginning to see more clearly the damage they do to themselves by adhering to the rigid stereotypes and demands of the male role. This is a critical time for mental health professionals to understand men's feelings and conflicts and to develop the most effective ways of helping men change in therapy. We hope this book will make a contribution toward moving us in this direction.

R. L. M., R. S. P.
B. G., J. A. A., L. B. F., S. G.

Acknowledgments

We wish to thank many people for their support and help in writing this book. First, we especially want to thank our collaborators for their insightful and sensitive contributions. We have truly enjoyed and been enriched by our joint effort. We also wish to thank Seymour Weingarten and Alan Gurman for their encouragement and editorial comments throughout this project.

Much of our inspiration for writing comes from our colleagues, supervisors, teachers, and friends who first raised our consciousness about the issue of gender in therapy, particularly the male dilemma. Our colleagues at the Ann Arbor Center for the Family and the University of Connecticut School of Family Studies have been especially helpful. Also, special thanks to Ann Hartman, Joan Laird, Claudia Bebko, and Jo Ann Krestan who read initial drafts of the manuscript.

Our wives, Melissa and Pat, have been instrumental in opening our eyes to many of the issues we have long ignored or been insensitive to due to our own gender conditioning. We thank them and our children (as well as the families of the contributors) for their patience and support.

We also want to thank Isabel Lin, Kathi Nelson, and Laurie Bresler for their administrative support in putting the book together. A special thanks goes to John Bacon, who has contributed editorial comments, ideas, and inspiration throughout—his writing skills have certainly been appreciated and integrated into much of our writing. We thank all of the men and women we have seen individually, in couples, families, and groups for what we learned through their efforts to grow and change.

Finally, we acknowledge and express our gratitude to each other, for the support and encouragement we have both experienced throughout this project. We value the caring friendship that has grown as a result of our work together.

RICHARD L. METH
ROBERT S. PASICK

Contents

PART I

UNDERSTANDING MEN IN U.S. SOCIETY

·1·

The Road to Masculinity

RICHARD L. METH

When I grow up to be a man
Will I dig the same things that turn me on as a kid;
Will I look back and say I wish I hadn't done what I did . . .
When I grow up to be a man.

BRIAN WILSON, 1964

WHAT IS MASCULINITY?

The attainment of manhood is both a unique and complex experience often misunderstood by the therapeutic community. As there are many facets of masculinity, we need to understand male development within social, psychological, legal, cultural, and ethnic frames of reference. What does it mean to be male? What are the myriad factors that determine men's development? What are the messages about masculinity that significantly influence the development of male identity? Finally, what are the specific affective and behavioral characteristics of being male that influence men individually and in their relationships?

These are questions that we believe underlie much of the challenge in working with men in any psychotherapeutic context. To work effectively with men, the clinician's initial task is to understand that most men are unaware of how little control they exercise over their lives. Being a male in our society has been viewed as a privilege, but if we closely examine the result of growing up male, we will see that it is a mixed privilege to grow up male because along with the advantages most men feel compelled to behave in ways that are self-destructive and harmful to others.

3

Why are men so consumed with work? Why is it that in the process of working excessively men can be ignorant of the destruction to themselves and their families? Once men begin to conform to the code of masculinity, they've agreed to a life-style that imposes strict rules and limits with little flexibility.

Like actors in a play, men are handed a script which they learn must be closely followed. As little boys they are not asked to review this script, nor are they given much opportunity to make suggestions for changing any part of it. While playwrights and directors may allow actors the freedom to modify a script to assure a better fit with the actor, men are not permitted the same freedom to improvise. Our culture's concept of masculinity produces a script that prescribes for men certain ways to think, feel, and behave as a male—anything else is viewed as "feminine" and unacceptable.

This chapter will attempt to examine not only the content of this script but, more importantly, its impact on men and their relationships. The clinician who works with men in any therapeutic setting must understand that this script places impossible binds on men, and a number of vignettes are used to help illustrate the conflictual dilemmas that result. The road to masculinity twists and turns through some difficult terrain—terrain that can take its toll on a man's well-being.

Masculinity is determined by a complex interplay of one's physical, psychological, and emotional development, interacting with surrounding social and cultural norms. It is a difficult task to describe what it means to be male, simply because of the inherent problems generalizing about any one group. Ethnicity has come to be recognized as an important yet often neglected component of one's character. While this has been, for the most part, a beneficial realization for the mental health community, there are those who take strong exception to stereotypical portrayals of anyone. There are, of course, bound to be gender differences and exceptions within any large group, which includes the male gender.

Still, in attempting to examine the nature of the male experience, some generalizations can be useful if their limitations are recognized. From many years of work with men in our clinical practice we have observed certain experiences and patterns of behavior common to the vast majority of men. For most men who have grown up in our society, messages have been provided to guide and direct them from boyhood to adolescence and onto adulthood. To say that these messages are merely "provided" belies the power of the socialization process that begins at a very early age. Our experience shows how these messages are "ingrained" in boys at a very young age.

What are boys taught about being male? Are boys today learning something different from what boys learned in earlier decades? Have the years really changed the way we are socializing boys in the 80's, especially in light of the Women's Movement? We find many of the men we have interviewed, both young and old, have been exposed to the traditional messages about manhood and, yet, would like to change some patterns they believe are disruptive, even destructive to their lives. With any kind of change, shedding traditional roles and behaviors one has learned and practiced from childhood is often an arduous battle, one that many find too difficult to continue.

Gender Role Socialization

Gender politics are deeply embedded in the fabric of American society and, thus, over the course of our psychological and social development, profoundly influence how we see ourselves as men and women. For most family therapists, context becomes inseparable from our work. Therapists must recognize not only how context influences our client's sense of manhood, but also what we define as masculine, based on what we have learned and experience as men; female therapists, must evaluate their lifetime experiences with men since that is part of what shapes their concept of masculinity. Throughout this book, we will come back to this notion of context, as it serves as a reference point in therapy for men.

Being male can be considered from a strictly biologically perspective; it can also include any characteristic defined by the society or culture as "masculine." The distinction between male "sex role" and "gender role" behavior has been explored extensively in recent years, and for good reason. Sex roles have been described as specific behaviors pertaining to one's biological make-up from birth. Differences in the reproductive function is the most common basis for delineating sex role behavior. Gender roles, on the other hand, are not biological but social constructions, creating powerful expectations designed to outline acceptable behavior for each sex. For our purposes in this book, the reader should assume that unless specified, the authors are addressing gender roles for men, not sex roles; that is, personality characteristics of men developed in accordance with the expectations of society and the particular culture in which a man was socialized.

From the many workshops the authors presented on men in therapy, we have found much confusion and frustration in the therapeutic community in working with men and gender issues. Some of this can be attributed to our different experiences as men or with men. We all hold our own beliefs on the nature of "manhood," based primarily upon what we have learned or been taught to believe. What results are powerful stereotypes of masculinity, stereotypes that we accept at an early age and that influence our behavior as men or our thoughts about men as women.

These stereotypes can be damaging. Goldberg (1976, 1979, 1983) was one of the first writers to warn men about the hazards encountered by the male socialization experience. One of the dangers, according to Goldberg, is that the external pressure to project a masculine image to the public often painfully conflicts with one's inner needs (which may traditionally be considered "feminine" needs).

A common scenario is that a man just learned he was refused a promotion at work, and returns to his desk feeling disappointed, hurt, and angry. When he encounters a few of his colleagues, it is clear to them from his appearance that he did not get the promotion. When several ask him what happened, he retreats, withdrawing into himself and unable to concentrate. He feels terrible and does not know what to do. When he considers expressing his thoughts to his friends, he immediately rejects this idea. Though he may not have been consciously aware of his motives, he learned at an early age that vocalizing one's feelings was something women did, that it was not a masculine trait.

The fear of femininity and feminine values are common results of male socialization (and concomitantly sexism). Farrell (1974), one of the early outspoken leaders of the Men's Movement, exposed the male socialization process as harmful by describing ten commandments of masculinity that lead men to destructive behavior. Although some may consider his a histrionic and personalized reaction to male gender socialization, Farrell's book is intended to provoke men to reevaluate aspects of their development that result in rigid and perilous life-styles.

As with any learned pattern of behavior, men find it easier to continue familiar habits. Pressure to resist change manifests itself not only within the individual, but also from close significant others, friends, co-workers, and even the media. Social and political changes that resulted from the emergence of the Women's Movement have created opposing pressures. The blueprints for manhood are in the process of change.

Many men are beginning to believe that some of what they have learned about being male profoundly interferes with the personal fulfillment they desire, especially in relationships with women. Men are buying books designed to challenge them, and to reassess the traditional concepts of manhood that alienate them from their feelings, and concomitantly, create circumstances ripe for self-destruction (Farrells, 1975; Goldberg, 1976). Books written especially for men in past years have generally offered the same message: The effort to pursue the success and achievement that they have been programmed for forces men to neglect and deny other needs that impede other kinds of success.

This is a common belief generally held by those who write for the nonprofessional audience. One needs only spend some time around a newstand and browse popular magazines. If we are to believe that the articles written about men reflect current trends, we can only conclude that men cannot love or experience closeness. They are either sexually demanding, clumsy, disinterested, or unable to consider a woman's sexual needs, they continually try to escape from relationships. This is a frequent complaint heard by marital therapists. Yet, according to a study by Pleck and Lang (1978), increasing numbers of men report that family and marital relationships are the most important things in their life, more so even than their careers.

Many of the therapists we have spoken with state that men now want to be more psychologically connected with their families; they desire more family activities and talk of achieving more fulfilling relationships than they had experienced growing up. So where do these desires meet reality? Do men feel? Do men have needs other than physical ones? Are men expressive, and do they desire to be emotionally close with another person? Are the articles in *Cosmopolitan*, *Ms.*, and similiar magazines a true depiction of the male gender, are they a slight distortion, or are these articles merely a sensationalized form of journalism designed to sell magazines? The answers are best addressed by carefully examining the process of male identity development. In the next section, we will look at the male experience from an early age to gain a better understanding of what shapes the male psyche.

MALE IDENTITY DEVELOPMENT

As we all know, there are no written guidelines that tell us how to behave as men or women. How we are to think, feel, and act as a member of a particular gender gets transmitted to us at an early age in more subtle forms and from a variety of sources. Recent studies of the effects of sex hormones on personality development suggest a genetic basis for some of the differences we observe between men and women (Treadwell, 1987). Yet this does not exclude other factors, and numerous contributions from social scientists effectively demonstrate the power of the socialization process (Balswick, 1971, 1977; Carrigan et al., 1987; O'Neil, 1982).

A man's expectations of himself are learned in boyhood, beginning almost from infancy, through contact with primary caretakers, significant others, and other persons who, though perhaps indirectly or unconsciously, influence the socialization process. It may be useful to think of this development in terms of various structures. For example, we know that a family can be viewed as a large structure containing many substructures (or subsystems) that have specific rules and guidelines as to how each substructure should function. As systems theory has evolved, an increasing proportion of emphasis has been placed on the importance of structures outside the family; in other words, clinicians broadened their view to include the macro-structures as they may have significant impact on the behavior of family members. Gender distinctions are reinforced by these larger structures, which prove to be highly influential forces on male identity development. Before we consider the effects of structures outside of the family, however, we need to assess early influences on male identity, influences that affect the rules which govern how males learn how to think, behave, and feel.

In a society where mothers continue to provide primary care and establish the most meaningful relationship for the infant, the sense of self that boys and girls develop typically evolves in relation to her. According to Chodorow (1978), the infant's dependence upon its mother for all of its emotional and physical needs creates a relational climate that exerts a powerful influence on the emerging gender identity. Chodorow's analysis, although firmly rooted in traditional psychoanalytic theory, offers a valuable perspective to view the early determinants of gender development, a perspective easily integrated into a system's model of therapy.

Chodorow's analysis skillfully combines the impact of the basic psychological processes and the individual's evolving psychic structures. For example, she examines the nature of the infant/mother attachment and elucidates distinctions that suggest that the nature of attachment is different for girls and boys. The oedipal triangle is one vehicle, according to Chodorow, that promotes a greater conflictual environment for the male infant, due to the competitive struggles which emerge later. This competitiveness, and the simultaneous struggle for identification with father (or other male figures), alters whatever stability had existed in the mother/child relationship. Compared to young girls, young males begin to experience the processes of attachment and separation in more unpredictable, discontinuous shifts. A girl, by contrast, remains more closely attached to the mother, which creates a degree of closeness rarely challenged by outside forces, including gender. According to Chodorow, this is a critical difference which provides the preconditions for some of the gender struggles that boys face later in their development.

Chodorow's analysis reveals that patterns of fusion, symbiosis, attachment, and separateness are different for men and women. Basically, the male infant's sense of connectedness with the primary caretaker becomes an ambivalent relationship, a delicate balance between his needs for a sense of emotional intimacy and the equally urgent need for identity, which leads to detachment and emotional distancing from the mother.

If we are to agree with Chodorow's theory, then we recognize how men struggle with their needs for both closeness and distance from a very early age. However, men rarely realize why these needs conflict. They often cannot articulate why they become emotionally detached, especially when they believe they want to feel closer. Men are at a loss to explain how they can desire a nurturing relationship yet create emotional distance and deny dependency. A man's struggle with intimate relationships may be attributed to processes that begin to occur at an age when they are barely cognizant of the subtle forces shaping their personalities.

Chodorow's perspective is important because it illustrates how boys and girls are influenced by gender prior to any socialization experience. It raises the question of gender role development. Is this the result of our society's rigid separation between men's and women's behavior, or do internalized subconscious images from real and imagined experiences precede whatever external influences follow?

Particularly relevant for the family therapist is the extent that gender composition influences and underlies shifts in family structure. When a boy pulls away from the close bond established with mother, the amount of emotional involvement and nurturing from father becomes a critical factor. If a boy's father is unable to provide some of nurturing lost by this separation, then the cycle of denial of emotional needs may be perpetuated to the next generation.

Another central element is the mother's treatment of the boy versus the girl infant. Although some researchers claim there is no behavioral evidence with parents to suggest any differential treatment (Maccoby & Jacklin, 1974), Chodorow currently states that the results are inconsistent, which suggests that one might find theoretical support for both positions. Again, generalizations are dangerous due to contextual differences such as race and ethnicity. Some cultures or socioeconomic groups may make it very clear that boys are to be treated differently than girls. For example, a college professor stated that in his family there was no distinction made between work assigned to his son or daughter. On the other hand, a line factory worker makes it very clear that he expects more from his son than his daughter, and does not assign "tough jobs" to her. Of course, his influence is only part of what impacts on his children's development.

There are numerous studies by sociologists and social psychologists which have demonstrated how sensitive young children, especially boys, are to distinctions made according to gender. Although too numerous to mention here, the conclusions are very similiar: As early as 3 and 4 years of age, boys are cognizant of what constitutes masculine behavior and what is considered feminine; they make efforts to prescribe to those toys and games that fall under the category of "masculine." One study asked boys and girls to label specific kinds of toys and games as "masculine" or "feminine" (Hartley, 1959). The author found that boys demonstrated and were able to make gender distinctions based on "appropriate" male behavior, whereas girls did not seem to have as rigid a sense of what games were considered "masculine" or "feminine." The results also revealed "the kinds of pressure young boys experience to be manly by adhering to certain sex-role standards" (p. 465). The implications of this study reinforce how socialization creates powerful gender distinctions that restrict the behavior of boys as they grow up.

Becoming a man entails learning not only what endeavors are consistent with being masculine, but what are considered feminine activities. As boys begin to consolidate their identity, they develop an acute sensitivity and ability to discriminate between masculine and feminine behavior, and typically avoid anything associated with femininity.

It is important to stress here that social and economic status, race, and ethnicity are all factors that affect how much young boys will attend to these gender role differences. This is where context becomes paramount. For example, a father of a 5-year-old boy discussed the kinds of toys he wanted his son to play with. Al, a 41-year-old physician, talked about deliberately trying to expose his son to toys that had been advertised to children along gender lines. He felt quite comfortable with his son playing with a doll (which he emphasized was his, not his sisters) as much as trucks and cars, which he also liked to play with. "I feel it is important that my son grows up learning how to be expressive in relationships, and doll play allows for more of this than with his trucks."

In contrast, Tom, a 34-year-old foreman in a print shop, responded to my question whether his 8-year-old son ever played with dolls this way: "You got to be kidding; there's no way I'd let my son do that, unless I wanted him to grow up to be like a girl. And if I ever did see him play with those kinds of girl toys, I'd take them right away from him. No way will he grow up to be the kind of man I think he should be if he plays with girl toys." I asked another father how he felt about taking his son to the Walt Disney movie, Snow White. Dan, a 37-year-old computer programmer for a large insurance company, was eager to talk about this subject. The question prompted him to recall his relationship with his father, which was quite distant. "No, I can never remember him taking me to the movies. It was always my mother. To me, the important thing is that my son and I go together . . . it doesn't matter whether it is to see Snow White or Star Wars, it's just the idea that we're doing something together . . ."

These men represent three disparate kinds of attitudes which are fairly common among men today, and certainly more prevalent than what existed 25 years ago. In the first two examples, Al and Tom respond with specific gender biases. Al is aware of the socialization process that boys experience and thus makes an effort to encourage activities which do not comply with gender role stereotypes. However, Tom may represent a greater percentage of fathers, although many men may not be as candid as Tom is in stating his fears of his son becoming effeminate. Dan is a man that most clinicians could surely sympathize with, in his attempt to provide his son with a relationship that he never had with his father. Consequently, issues of gender are secondary for him. Do we really believe that for men like Dan the importance of quality relationship overshadows what he has learned about gender through his own socialization? Much of the literature on men and gender roles refutes this.

Researchers who examine the process of male socialization have identified a number of powerful underlying forces responsible for male gender bias. One most frequently cited in the literature is a man's distrust or fear of femininity. This fear of appearing feminine often is responsible for the way men act, feel, and behave (Balswick, 1979; O'Neil, 1981). Many conclude that being "masculine" is equivalent to not doing the kinds of things one would expect a woman to do.

The experts who write about male socialization generally agree that men avoid any behaviors or mannerisms that could be construed as "feminine." What does this mean, then, in a practical sense? For example, let's say that a boy grows up with the message that "big boys don't cry," and, consequently, he rarely expresses sadness, even later in life. Playing with dolls is another example. Because this is frequently viewed as something only girls do, boys tend to avoid any kind of behavior that even resembles such play. One 6-year-old boy I recently asked about this gave me a very straight answer, "It's boring; that's why I don't play with dolls. Anyway, dolls are for girls." One aspect of "contemporary manhood," therefore, seems to be avoiding feminine behavior. Yet, this does not complete the question, what does it mean to be a male?

Male Power: Privilege or Burden?

In political systems throughout history, men have generally been sole owners of the power. Until recently, few have looked at how this imbalance of power affects our daily lives. Those who have studied and examined the male use of power provide compelling evidence of the exploitation and abuse of power by men not only in our society but throughout the world (Henley, 1977; Lipman-Blumen, 1984). Lipman-Blumen (1984) states, "Great effort has been devoted towards preserving these polarized differences, which symbolize the power differential between male and female gender roles in most societies" (p. 5). She maintains that the need for power is frequently a response to the uncertainty and anxiety generated by living in an environment humans have little capacity to control. Therefore, the power relationship is one means by which men can convince themselves they have some control over part of their environment.

In an effort to increase public awareness of the power imbalance in our society, the Feminist Movement exposed and questioned the uses and abuses of male power (Polk, 1974). Confronting the disadvantages of being rendered powerless encouraged women to challenge and change the subordinate position delegated to them by our patriarchical society. Inspired by the Women's Movement, others pointed out that men have used their power not only to subordinate but to devalue and ignore the accomplishments of women (Massengill & Di Marco, 1979), while continuing to abuse women physically and emotionally (Roy, 1977).

Women's voices began to be heard. As the "power war" progressed, men had to face a diminished realm of power, status, and control over women in the home and workplace. Those who researched the male response to such power loss affirmed the message of the feminists. Kahn noted that "male power, especially over females, appears to be central to many men's definitions of themselves. With power they are men; without it they are no better than women" (Kahn, 1984, p. 238). For some men, however, possessing power may not be any more advantageous than not having it.

According to one author, the reality is that men have surprisingly little autonomy or power (Astrachan, 1986). While some men may view women as dependent, powerless, or the weaker sex, men, too, are limited in their choices. The confines of the male gender role offer only a narrow range of behaviors which allow a man access to external rewards, but do not, as Farrell (1986) observes, lead to control over his own life. He concluded that men actually have very little power, if power is redefined as autonomy over one's own life. Farrell believes, for example, that the external rewards and benefits that men gain from positions of authority (which includes power and status) seldom satisfy their expectations. Inner peace, emotional expression, affection, sexual fulfillment, and physical health are areas that men frequently have little control over due to the constraints of male socialization.

Men learn to devalue, or at least deny, the need for internal rewards (Farrell, 1986). For men, emotional support and nurturing connote weakness. Although men may appear powerful on the outside, many are unable to alter the internal side effects. The statistics on the differences in males' and females' physical health demonstrate how destructive this mind-set can be for men. Not only do women live 7.8 years longer than men, men suffer over 98% of the major diseases (U.S. Bureau of Census, 1984, p. 79). The aggressive pursuit of power may produce prestige, authority, and money, but men rarely are aware of or even consider the negative consequences. External power frequently leads to self-neglect.

Power, aggression, and restraint are traits that have long been associated with male behavior. As a concept central to contemporary masculinity, the importance of power dates back to the early caveman and hunter. Men were expected to be powerful and successful hunters in order to provide the necessary supplies for their family; aggression and physical strength were vital to fulfill this role. In factories and mines, where much of the labor required physical strength, men occupied most of the jobs. This was no different for the farm family. The division of labor on the farm was typically broken down by men taking on most of the work outside of the home. Once a man walked inside after a days work, his job was over until the next day.

In the past, people did not question this hierarchy, which provided certain rewards for men. If men worked hard during the day, they felt they deserved to relax when they returned home. Furthermore, this sense of entitlement was derived in part from their status as the family's sole breadwinner. Before the emergence of the dual career family, this arrangement was rarely challenged by families in the United States.

The social structure of the time not only reinforced the allotment of work according to gender, it also strengthened many stereotypes of "men's work" and "women's work," which coincided with similar biases of "male" and "female" behavior. Men and women were given well-delineated guidelines for appropriate actions, thoughts, and feelings. Masculinity and femininity fell at opposite ends of the behavioral continuum and offered little room for flexibility. When a man had qualities labeled "feminine," he would clearly feel his sense of self and identity as a man were threatened. Because this gender dichotomy presented little middle ground, men could choose only from those behaviors that were perceived as decidedly masculine. This was perhaps best demonstrated by Levinson's research in the late 1970s.

Masculinity–Femininity: A Restrictive Dichotomy

Levinson et al. (1978) provide direct support to the notion that men carefully and systematically avoid feminine behavior. They found that almost all of the men in their sample experienced a masculine/feminine polarity that caused varying degrees of conflict, depending on the man's age, marital status, and vocation. To explore this in more detail, Levinson et al. asked men to explain what they associated with each gender. According to the men interviewed, being masculine meant the following:

1. Having power, exercising control over others, and being and recognized as being a leader (one of strong will).
2. Having strength, toughness, and stamina, and able to endure bodily stress.
3. Logical and analytical in thought, and intellectually competent.
4. High achievement and ambition to be successful in their work.

Men were also asked to describe their conceptions of femininity. The characteristics considered feminine were as follows:

1. Weakness, frailty, submissiveness, and unassertive behavior; limited bodily resources; vulnerable to exploitation.
2. Decisions based on emotions and intuition, rather than on careful analysis.
3. Nurturing disposition, including taking care of others' (husband, children) needs.
4. Homosexuality.

Levinson's data are reflected in other studies on male identity. David and Brannon (1976) also list power, control, toughness, and ambition as major components of male sex-role development. They entitle the first section of their book *The Forty-Nine Percent Majority*, which presents the dimensions of the male sex role, "No Sissy

Stuff: The Stigma of Anything Vaguely Feminine." In their introduction, David and Brannon state that the fear of femininity produces "guidelines" as to how a "real man" should carry himself. Furthermore, they believe that a man's "aura of toughness" may be a compensatory measure for men to avoid feminine behavior. To be tough is to deny vulnerability and project strength, even when one feels weak.

A man experiences any particular facet of the self that he considers feminine with great conflict and anxiety, because he believes it threatens his manhood. Consequently, the costs of exhibiting "feminine qualities" are paid in lowered self-esteem, self-concept, and masculine identity. Over time, men learn to selectively incorporate behaviors that will enhance their male self-image; similarly, men systematically discard qualities that are seen as predominantly feminine. It should be emphasized that this process, usually not a conscious one, evolves over a lifetime of exposure to signals our society repeatedly provides.

Emotional expressiveness, a trait typically associated with being feminine, presents a good example of this. Emotionally expressive individuals can vent a wide range of feelings, both verbally and nonverbally. This consequently gives them an inner awareness and connection to their feelings. Once individuals develop this familiarity with their feelings, they can more readily choose which ones to express and which not to express, thus gaining mastery over emotions.

Do men have the ability to connect with their feelings, and then relate these feelings to others? Are men aware of the range of emotions that are triggered by events in their daily lives? Do men deliberately pick and choose which feelings they will acknowledge and express. Finally, how conscious is this process? Obviously there are no simple answers to these questions. Yet if our clinical experience is any indication, it would be difficult to argue against the powerful forces of socialization, which many writers believe not only create the male gender role but are also responsible for the self-destructive behavior that results from adherence to gender-role prescriptions (Balswick & Peek, 1971; Farrells, 1974; Goldberg, 1976; Lewis, 1978; O'Neil, 1982; Pleck, 1976; Skovholt, 1978).

Physical intimacy with other men is something men typically avoid at all costs due to homophobia and mens' fears of femininity.

This fear of femininity has been described in great detail (Balswick & Peek, 1971; Bear, Berger, & Wright, 1979; David & Brannon, 1976; Harrison, 1978; Levison et al., 1978; Lewis, 1978; O'Neil, 1982; Pleck, 1976; Skovholt, 1978). Homophobia, the fear of being, becoming, or having any traits or qualities characteristic of homosexuals, has also been addressed in several books (Lehne, 1976; O'Neil, 1981). These fears, often unconscious yet powerful, result in many rules that regulate acceptable physical intimacy around men. For many cultures, "real men" must not possess any feminine characteristics, which can be numerous. Yet in some selective cultures and ethnic groups, physical affection is viewed as acceptable and expected behavior from men, especially in the ritual of greeting or saying goodbye. It is beyond the scope of this chapter to pursue this in greater detail, but those interested in reading about cultural differences can read the text *Ethnicity and Family Therapy*, by McGoldrick et al. (1982)—a valuable resource.

Avoiding all behavior associated with being feminine can create gender-role strain and conflict. O'Neil (1982) described six patterns of gender role strain and conflict including (1) restrictive emotionality, (2) homophobia, (3) socialized control, power and competitive issues, (4) restricted sexual and affectionate behaviors, (5) obsession with achievement and success, and (6) health problems. Pleck (1982) made the connection between the narrow range of behaviors men allow themselves within the male gender role and the subsequent sex-role strain. Pleck (1981) found that society has constructed a psychology of masculinity based on myths and assumptions about men that is now deeply embedded within the social structure of our society. This male sex-role identity (MSRI) paradigm, which has been learned and incorporated into our society since the early 1900s, guides male behavior by dictating what is acceptable for men to think, feel, and do. Although some theorists make a clear distinction between sex role and gender role, Pleck (1981) uses these concepts interchangably in describing the sex-role strain (SRS) model.

Sex-role strain results when men attempt to adhere to prescribed behaviors and limit other behaviors that may be useful at certain times. In other words, certain characteristics developed from sex or gender roles can become psychologically dysfunctional. For example, according to the MSRI paradigm, men have internalized powerful images and beliefs regarding self-disclosure. These images, many resulting from messages within the family, manifest the expression of feelings as a feminine trait, which reveals vulnerability and weakness. What happens when men violate this code and express emotion openly? An apt example is the one presented earlier of the man who failed to get the promotion he had waited for, for so long.

One could expect this man to experience a range of emotions, some of which he might feel more permission to express as a man, such as anger and resentment. But what about the hurt and rejection he felt? He considers carefully what would happen if he expressed these feelings, since to express hurt or rejection may reveal weakness, but he feels that the decision was grossly unjust, and decides to go to management to fight for his promotion. During this discussion, feelings surface, which he vents openly, even tearing up at one point. Several days later, his boss recommends that he take some time off since he is so upset. His boss also tells him that the promotion would have brought him stress and more work, something his boss thought he could not handle. While staying within the confines of male gender roles can be restrictive, behaving in ways not sanctioned within the code of male gender roles can also have damaging effects.

AFFECTIVE AND BEHAVIORAL DIMENSIONS OF MASCULINITY

Men learn there are specific affective and behavioral dimensions to being male. The rules learned growing up as a man serve as blueprints that govern how men will behave. Within the affective domain the message is clear: Men should not express anything that makes them appear vulnerable and should be careful to express only what they consider safe. The result is that many men eschew any form of emotional expression that may connote femininity. However, among women, men may not be as careful to conceal their emotions. Michael, a 36-year-old school psychologist, describes how his relations with women differ from those with men.

> "It is amazing to me how different my conversations are with women. This is especially true in the teachers' lounge at work. If I'm talking with the guys, it's usually about sports or something macho. While I'm involved in this discussion, I overhear women in the room talking

about stuff that goes on in their relationships and I feel jealous. Then I realize, I can't talk about this stuff here, not with these guys. They'd probably laugh at me or make me out to be like some woman. But then I think, what would the guys think if I excused myself to go talk with the women. I end up leaving the guys to talk with the women, and, believe it or not, I find their discussions more interesting."

Michael's testimony exposes the quintessential male dilemma, one where men weigh the benefit of emotional expression against the risks of self-exposure. His decision to not disclose his personal feelings to his male peers was a conscious one, but for many men, this process usually occurs without any conscious awareness. Regardless, this decision has important implications for the kind of intimacy men can experience in any relationship. Of course, we first must understand the male view of intimacy.

Not surprisingly, many men associate intimacy with sex. Does this mean that men only desire intimacy in conjunction with sexuality? Have men learned or been permitted to be intimate in other ways?

Ask a male client about his idea of intimacy. You might find that many men have difficulty answering the question from their own perspective, rather than their partner's. But, some responses might eventually appear. "Intimacy is sharing your experiences," says one man. "Intimacy means knowing that someone cares about you as much as you care about them," says another. Marty expressed his confusion about intimacy this way:

> "I can never quite understand what you people mean by intimacy. According to my standards, I feel pretty good about my relationship with my wife. We do things together, we have a decent sexual relationship (although it could be better), I tell her about my day when I get home. But it doesn't seem to be enough for her. She complains that I don't talk to her about my real feelings. That's when I get really pissed off. I mean, I tell her what's on my mind, what more does she want from me? And then, she thinks that all I want is sex, like I'm some kind of sex maniac or something. I like touching my wife, but she reacts like I'm doing something dirty. Sometimes I wonder that maybe she doesn't like sex. I don't know, it's just very frustrating to know what will make her happy."

The frustration expressed by Marty is not unique. He has discovered the awkwardness so many men experience in their attempt to become intimate with their partner, a struggle Rubin (1983) describes as the "approach–avoidance dance." Contrary to what some may think, men want and need what an intimate relationship can offer. Men raised in our society, however, learn to restrict self-expression. Marty's view of himself as a sex maniac can only lead to increased feelings of inadequacy and failure as he struggles to feel like a competent husband. What does Marty need to learn to overcome his dilemma?

As we know, men are taught to control their emotions. In addition to the messages that encourage men to be reticent, however, are rules that dictate appropriate physical contact. The process of weaning from the primary caretaker, discussed earlier from Chodorow's perspective, continues throughout childhood. Young boys gradually have less physical contact with their mother, because they sense that it is expected of them. Even in situations where a young boy experiences particularly intense pain and discomfort, such as the death of a family member, he is encouraged to be strong, take care of himself, and be available when others might need him.

Unlike adolescent girls, who are encouraged to express physical affection with one another, boys the same age are unlikely to express themselves with male peers in similiar ways. Except for the congratulatory pat on the back during an athletic event, boys will usually eschew any kind of physical contact. In fact, most boys have virtually no physical contact of any kind until they begin to date and experiment sexually. Touching and physical affection become synonomous with sex. It is no surprise then that as the adolescent male develops into young adulthood, intimate experiences are often associated with sexual activity.

On an affective level, men are only encouraged to express what is permissible according to the rules of masculinity. Since they are conditioned to persistently avoid behaving in feminine ways, men often appear to be devoid of feelings. Nevertheless, men have undeniable needs for which they must find an acceptable outlet.

Sex can be the sole vehicle of intimacy for men. For men like Marty, sex becomes the most familiar, spontaneous, and acceptable way to experience intimate feelings. But does this mean Marty need not learn new ways of being intimate? In evaluating Marty's situation, context is again an important consideration. Here it is the 1980s, a time that follows a decade, and more, of men and women questioning and changing the assumptions of traditional male behavior.

MEN IN TRANSITION: MEN IN THE 90'S

Are men shedding the burden of traditional male roles? Do men even view or experience these traditional roles as burdens? When analyzing men in transition we must remind ourselves that we are not addressing the concerns of all men or perhaps even most men. More likely, it is only a small group of men who are conscious of their struggle with conflicting messages of manhood. Men who find themselves in the psychotherapist's office are not always there to change their role orientation. So, who are the men who are ready to challenge what they have been taught?

In my experience there are not large numbers of men entering therapy due to conflicts over gender roles. This is not to say that gender-role conflict is not an issue for many men. But therapists may prematurely present gender issues to men even when they are not ready to acknowledge it is problematic for them. The results are predictable:

Emile, 41, and Ronnie, 40, his wife, entered marital therapy following a fight where both struck physical blows. As they recounted the events that led up to the incident, it was clear that Emile used his size and his greater earning capacity as leverage in their relationship. The therapist, recognizing the power unbalance as one source of dysfunction, decided to immediately address the gender issues and Emile's need to control. When the therapist (who was male) asked Emile to consider these issues, Emile became defensive, stating that no one was going to tell him how he should act. Sensing that the husband may have felt he was siding with the wife, the therapist backed off. Another session was scheduled, but the following day the wife called to say her husband would not come back.

John was referred to treatment after meeting with a counselor in the company's employee assistance program. Although he considered himself only a "social drinker," his frequent binges caused him to miss many days of work. Although he followed the counselor's suggestion to see a therapist, he did this only to protect his job. He was not surprised when the therapist identified his drinking as a major problem to be worked on. Yet, he resented the therapist who suggested he should stop drinking. He decided he would go to therapy a couples of times to appease his supervisor but thought to himself that no one had the right to tell him to stop drinking. A month later, after missing three days of work, he was fired. When the therapist suggested that his alcohol use may still be a problem, John vehemently denied this had anything to do with his job loss. He called his therapist to cancel his next appointment "because he no longer needed it."

Earlier in this chapter we mentioned the Men's Liberation Movement, which is not of the same magnitude as the Feminists' Movement. The numbers involved are not as great as the Women's Movement, and there has not been the same level of commitment and organization. Nevertheless, there has been an outpouring of literature that clearly expresses the dilemmas men reared on traditional roles are experiencing. A number of the so-called "male liberationists," mostly men in the mental health field, have begun to publish books for those men who are prepared to reevaluate themselves. Some books have addressed the "male transition" (Dubbert, 1979; Farrell, 1974; Nichols, 1975), while others analyze the myth of masculinity and male temperament (Kriegel, 1978; La Haye, 1977), the hazards of being male (Goldberg, 1976), and male intimacy (Naifeh & Smith, 1984). One man's struggle resulted in a book entitled *The Men's Survival Book: Being a Man in Today's World* (Cooke, 1975), which might be considered evidence of the incredible stress some men experience from these changes. Women who want to find a resource in understanding men could refer to *Men: A Book for Women* (Wagenvoord & Bailey, 1978) for insight and direction.

In the past 10 to 15 years, men have been inundated with mandates to change from the media and significant others. Many authors have encouraged men to "tune in" to their bodies and pay more attention to indications of physical disorder and stress, especially in the workplace. Is success worth the price? What are the effects of the masculine role on mens' health? There is a consensus among these writers that some aspects of the traditional male role have a pernicious effect on mens' physical and psychological well-being.

Men, Sexuality, and the Changing Roles of Men

These days women are less likely to allow men alone to define their sexual relationship. The new climate of sexual openness challenges the traditional balance of men's sexual autonomy. The Feminist Movement encourages women to talk more freely to their partners about their own sexuality. However, the positive changes women make are not always received as improvements by men.

A recent study suggests that the new shifts of gender relations have increased the frequency of male impotence (Gould, 1982). The difficult relational dynamics outside of the bedroom can have deleterious effects inside the bedroom for men. Stephen, a 33-year-old computer consultant, described himself as "always ready for sex." Since becoming sexually active at age 18, Stephen had always enjoyed sexual relationships with women. He married Karen when he was 27 and she was 25. For the first 2 years the couple's sexual relationship was "mutually satisfying," with both free to initiate sexual contact. But something began to change, according to Stephen:

> "Things were great for the first couple of years; even after the baby was born our sexual relationship continued to be enjoyable to both of us. But then Karen went back to work and somehow we both seemed to lose interest in sex. Actually, I hate to admit it, but it was more me. I think I resented her job. She would come home and tell me about her day and . . . I would start to get real depressed and resentful. Why? . . . I'm not sure. Maybe deep down I am angry about the job she went back to. It pays well and, of course, we need the money, but the idea of my wife making more money than I do bothers me more than I realize. I'm supposed to be the breadwinner and support my family. But we can't make it on just my salary. It's funny because my father made a lot less than I do; yet I can't imagine him letting my mother go to work; his ego wouldn't allow anything like that."

Fred, a 41-year-old lawyer, was referred for psychotherapy, after consulting his family physician for impotence which had continued for several months. His wife, Catherine, age 40, called the therapist to make the appointment because Fred refused. After many false starts, Fred came in to talk. When I asked him if he had any ideas of what caused his sexual dysfunction, he said:

> "I don't know what happened, but things have not been clicking with us. I always thought I had satisfied Catherine, but . . . she started saying things during sex which just seemed to throw me. In the ten years we have been married I had thought she had been satisfied with me as a lover. I was a lot more experienced than Catherine, and figured I knew what she needed as a woman. So you could just imagine how I felt when she told me she had not really enjoyed what I had been doing during lovemaking. At first, I blamed her therapist, thinking she was putting these ideas in her head. But then she told me that she had not been happy for a long time; she said that it was her therapy that helped her realize this. Now that I look back, there were signals, but I

didn't pick up on them. Maybe I just didn't want to hear what she was trying to tell me. Anyway, the problem still continues. Catherine thinks that the impotence is an ego thing. I think that's ridiculous; it's probably something physical. As a matter of fact, I have an appointment with the urologist tomorrow."

Fred erroneously believes the myth that a man is a good lover by instinct, that he does not learn but should already know a variety of techniques that will satisfy any woman. Although traditional sexual rules have been replaced with more egalitarian approaches, not all men are aware of or receptive to these new values. For men, much of their masculine identity is embedded in their performance, and sexual performance is no exception.

Earlier, we discussed the male preoccupation with achievement and performance. This is true for adolescent males, who are also preoccupied with sexuality. Boys discover that their private feelings about anything sexual become public domain. There is a code outlining what boys are expected to divulge. From their peer group, the message is that they are to report every aspect of their sexual behavior, from their first kiss to their first intercourse (viewed by some as a "conquest"). Some boys also engage in group masturbation as a means of testing their sexual apparatus and demonstrating that it works to their friends and themselves. Boys often like to boast about any kind of sexual activity, in part to inform their peers of their progress but also as a means of validating their emerging manhood. Yet there is an old locker room theory that holds that the one who brags the most about sexual encounters is generally the one who has actually had the fewest.

Just as much as men want to feel successful as sexual partners, they fear failure and incompetence. As a result, men often exaggerate the extent of their sexual experience and knowledge. I am reminded of a memorable scene of the John Hughes' movie, *Sixteen Candles*. Molly and Michael have both left the dance, and are sitting in a car discussing the awkwardness of adolescence. Molly has just told Michael something very personal, and feels quite vulnerable. Michael recognizes this, turns to her, and says:

MICHAEL: O.K., I'll tell you something about me, but you have to promise never to tell anyone, because if you do, it will totally ruin my reputation as a dude . . . (Molly nods her head and promises not to reveal this deep, dark secret.) I never bagged a babe. (Molly reacts with laughter and surprise.) Well I'm sorry, excuse me for being a virgin." (Michael appears to regret telling Molly this painful truth no one else knows.)

MOLLY: "I'm not laughing at you . . . It's just, well, what's so bad about that . . . I'm a virgin too.

Achievement-oriented sexual pressures do not seem to affect girls in the same way. For boys, loss of virginity is a rite of passage that must be experienced in order to feel like one is developing normally. Yet it is important to remember that these pressures may be more characteristic of the male adolescent in the United States than adolescents in other cultures. Other cultures may not subtly pressure adolescent boys to become sexually active so soon. In fact, some cultures encourage suppression of sexual impulses until the young male is ready to marry. The case of Alex, an 18-year-old Russian immigrant, reveals what happens when someone with a different sexuality enters an American male adolescent peer group:

Alex was referred to the mental health clinic by his family physician for a "sexual problem." He told the therapist how difficult it was for him to come for therapy, but the discomfort was so great, according to Alex, he could no longer ignore the problem. Basically, Alex was afraid to get involved with any woman. A very handsome and well-built individual, Alex had been co-captain of his high school soccer team. Now, in his freshman year at college, he was being pursued by numerous young women attracted to this new campus sensation. Whether in a bar or at a party, he would become overwhelmed with anxiety at the thought of being with a woman sexually. He usually found some reason to excuse himself from wherever he was so he could avoid this kind of contact. And while he had not wanted to call attention to himself, people began to notice his avoidance behavior. Finally, even his best male friends began to ask questions.

A fairly detailed psychosocial developmental history did not reveal anything particularly significant. But in the course of describing his transition to the United States, Alex talked about his experience living in the New York City area. It wasn't until the next session that he felt comfortable enough with me to reveal his reactions to the X-rated movies he had gone to numerous times with other recent Soviet immigrants.

When asked to describe how these movies affected him, Alex became a bit agitated. He had never seen such explicit sexual activity, and had found the movies both stimulating and frightening. What was most frightening, according to Alex, was "watching the men able to continue to perform repeatedly without losing their erection . . . and at how large their erections were . . .". Further discussion revealed that Alex had concluded he could never satisfy a woman the way these men did in the movies he had watched. This proved to be a turning point for therapy, as Alex now understood what was underlying his avoidance behavior and could work on dispelling the super-stud myths he had created.

The men described above obviously do not represent all of the problems men have with their sexuality; later chapters of this book address other sexual issues with which men struggle. The above examples attempt to explicate how a man's sense of himself is so inextricably bound to his sexual performance. Male gender-role development also significantly affects men's approach to physical health and illness. At this point, we will examine how the male gender role encourages ignoring signs of failing health.

Men and Physical Health

Just as men learn to deny emotions, they also learn to disregard any indication of bodily malfunction. In this regard, Goldberg (1976) believes that men's denial is so prevalent that it is one of the reasons their average life span is shorter than women's. Because men associate physical illness with vulnerability and weakness, they typically are reluctant to acknowledge pain or a symptom that could be life-threatening (Solomon, 1981). Even if he has experienced something as serious as a heart attack, denial may still prevail. The following story of Ted is an example of how denial distorts men's assessment of their physical well-being:

> Roberta, a consultation liason nurse in a large teaching hospital, was used to having her lunch interrupted. She called the paging operator, who connected her with the head nurse on the cardiac intensive care unit. The voice of the head nurse did not reflect the usual calm and competent manner she typified; with this call, her voice was strained and shaky, reflecting the crisis on her unit.
>
> Roberta arrived on the unit, unprepared for what was to come. Accustomed to seeing almost anything due to the nature of her job, she stood aghast in the hospital room, unable to believe what she was seeing. The

patient, a 35-year-old man who up until a few days ago worked regular shifts as an inner city cop and was now hospitalized on the cardiac intensive care unit for a massive heart attack, was jumping rope with the cord from the heart monitor device that had been keeping him alive.

Minutes earlier, several nurses from the cardiac unit attempted unsuccessfully to restrain the patient; Ted emphatically told the entire nursing team that as long as he had to stay in the hospital he was going to stay in shape, since his job required it. He mumbled something about maintaining his strength while they did "tests" on him. The nurse consultant, knowing the urgency and danger of the situation, searched for the right thing to say, realizing that every minute Ted continued this behavior posed more danger. In a voice as firm and as strong as she could muster, she demanded that Ted stop playing with the monitor cord before he broke the machine, since he would be responsible for paying for any damages. And she pointed out, his insurance would not cover for this; it would have to come out of his own pocket. He stopped when he realized that his insurance would not cover any damages to the expensive equipment he was abusing.

Ted's denial of his vulnerable state was clearly life-threatening. But as Goldberg (1976) points out, boys learn early that it is unmasculine to complain about illness. Again, the message is clear: A man preoccupied or even concerned with physical malfunctions is weak and therefore "unmanly." Although Ted's story may be an extreme case, strong denial is a common trait of most men, and places them at risk from the time they are very young.

Any practitioner who works with men soon discovers that they have an answer for everything, even when it comes to explaining or rationalizing health problems. As men learn to deny emotional and physical pain, they develop methods which insulate them from their pain. Rationalization, intellectualization, and logical thinking are three defenses that men use with considerable expertise. Of course, the potential hazard in developing these defenses as a skill is that it can lead to an abusive and self-destructive life style.

Typically, if a man is not expressive in the affective domain, his method of expression is intellectualizing—that is, he discusses his feelings in a detached and rational manner. This man can "feel great" one day and have a heart attack the next. This is the man who is frequently told how tired he looks, but does not go to bed early because he doesn't feel tired. This is the man who ignores the pain from a sports-related injury yet complains that he is not performing the way he usually does. Basically, this is a man who cannot hear the myriad signals his body attempts to send him.

Men who intellectualize their illness also fail to distinguish between different bodily symptoms. If a man experiences gastric distress and is also chronically tired, he might not see any potential relationship between the two. Suggest a possible connection, and he immediately dismisses it. Ron, a 45-year-old design engineer for a large government weapons contractor, is a good example of this dilemma:

> Ron was referred by his family physician after a complete physical exam revealed a developing gastritis condition accompanied by a generally run-down state of health. Initially, Ron was resistant to coming in because in his words he "couldn't afford to take the time off from a project which had to be completed in 3 weeks." As it turns out, this deadline was self-imposed and unrealistic, but nevertheless done to impress his boss and earn in his words "brownie points towards his promotion." I learned later on that Ron had been given 3 months to complete this assignment due to the complexity of the design.
>
> Because of his self-imposed pressure, Ron decided to work at home until late. This required him to drink 3 to 4 cups of coffee per night, in addition to the 2 to 4 cups of coffee he drank during the work day. He was sleeping only 5 to 6 hours per night instead of the 7 hours he was used to. Although family, co-workers, and friends noticed how tired and run down he appeared, Ron brushed off their concerns with an "I'm OK, don't worry about me" response. Instead of sitting down to dinner with his family he would retreat to his office to work, insisting he wasn't hungry. The seriousness of the situation was finally evident to his wife when she discovered several empty bottles of Maalox in the trash can of her husband's office. When confronted with this, Ron admitted that he had been having severe stomach pains for several weeks, but dismissed them as being "the least of his worries." In therapy, Ron began to look at the implications of his denial and the effects it was having on his work, family, and health.

Part of a man's resistance to acknowledging illness may be due to his fear of dependence on women as caretakers. Moreover, the assumption of dependency as feminine poses a threat to manhood. Although some men consider it unmasculine and therefore unacceptable to say they have dependency needs, for other men becoming ill can be a legitimate way of fulfilling dependency needs. However, the feeling of dependency that illness brings can also generate anxiety which potentially becomes more disabling than the illness itself. This anxiety can be brought on by the unplanned changes that occur in the delicate balance of intimacy in a relationship, especially for men who fear they will be engulfed by their partner to the point of smothering if they show any dependency.

Models of masculinity have implicitly instructed men to ignore diet, alcohol intake, amount of sleep needed, and emotional stress because of the supposed link to femininity (Nathanson, 1977). For those men who can transcend these fears of femininity, there is the opportunity to overcome some of the self-destructive behaviors men unknowingly engage in. Ironically, men who are consumed with the pursuit of success may not live long enough to enjoy the fruition of their labor. This was expressed most poignantly by David, a 51-year-old executive referred to therapy by his family physician.

David told the story of how his obsession with reaching the top almost resulted in his untimely death. Unknowingly, David would completely detach himself from his debilitating physical state, ignoring signals such as persistant shortness of breath when climbing the stairs at home. It was David's wife who intervened after hearing him become winded after climbing the stairs to a restaurant. Once confronted, David first tried to rationalize the symptoms as being related to smoking more heavily. Not totally convinced, David's wife scheduled him for a visit to the cardiologist. It was following a comprehensive cardiac work-up that David learned that one of his major arteries was blocked. To his surprise and to his wife's horror, the cardiologist recommended immediate bypass surgery as the only option that would save his life. Sitting in my office several months after surgery, David reflected on the massive denial that almost led to his death:

> "It was a shock, alright. I had no idea the problem was so bad. I guess what scares me the most is that I was so totally oblivious to what was going on inside my body. How stupid of me! But I never really payed too much attention to things like that. I never give myself a day at home; it was always the bank first, my family second, me last. And besides, I've known guys who were real hypochondriacs—you know, Woody Allen types—guys I wouldn't want to give a promotion to. All my life I've tried not to let little aches and pains get in my way. Like I used to pride myself on never missing a day of work. Anyway, now I

look at myself and guess I'm pretty lucky. Now I realize that all my pushing to get to the top is not worth it if it means not being around for my wife and children."

While David's first response is typical of many men who persist in denying illness, he is different in that he responded to his wife's concerns and went to see his doctor. There are men who may never respond to their wife's intervention as David did. These are the men who may also not live long enough to see their life dreams become reality.

Final Thoughts About Male Conditioning

This chapter has examined the many facets of masculinity, emphasizing the social and emotional impact of being male in our society. Gender roles have been and continue to be a major influence on how men think, feel, and behave. To work with men in any psychotherapeutic context, one must have a reasonable understanding of why men do what they do. With this perspective, we can develop ways of intervening in the lives of men who have been hampered by the process of male gender-role socialization. This stress can take on different forms at different points in a man's life.

The critical issues of male behavior vary at each stage of development. Young boys are encouraged to compete in games that require the expression of aggression and violence, whereas expression of other emotions is often discouraged. As young men face the demands and challenges of young adulthood, career choice and finding a mate become two central concerns, and gender roles continue to bear heavily on their well-being. Adolescent males have a number of developmental tasks unique to their stage of life, although these tasks have no clear-cut beginning or end. As young men grow up, they become precisely attuned to the masculine behavior expected of them.

Caught between conflicting desires, young men often struggle to succeed in the different roles they take on. Finding a reasonable balance is difficult. This manifests itself once a man establishes himself in a career, while attempting to maintain a commitment to his family. The need to be successful, forever prevalent and typically measured by how much money one can make, can interfere with familial objectives.

Most men in all age groups, grow up feeling tremendous anxiety about intimacy, in part due to the dependency and vulnerability that surface in close relationships. This places some men in a highly conflicted state, where they may often experience profound frustration and failure. Ironically, this frustration prompts men to invest less in relationships and more in work, where they may feel they have a better chance for success. Although finding some kind of balance in life is clearly important to reduce stress, for many men this is an emphemeral phenomenon. This will be discussed in greater depth in the second part of this book.

Middle age presents a new set of concerns. During these years men will reflect and evaluate their accomplishments. Did they fulfill their life dreams? Have they been a success in their job? Is their family life one that provides satisfaction? Do they love their wife? Do they stay in their marriage?

Because of the ingrained tendency to avoid feelings of vulnerability, men may not respond directly to the emotional turmoil that the middle years generate. Unable to deal directly with feelings of inadequacy or failure, middle-aged men may turn to new relationships or business ventures, with little regard for the negative consequences of their behavior.

During the later years, men must come to terms with declining physical health and strength, whereas good physical health and strength may have been a source of gratification and achievement in their younger years. Earlier conflicts with dependency resurface as men need to turn to others more frequently in middle age and, in some instances, allow themselves to be taken care of.

Some men may meet early deaths due to many of the self-destructive tendencies they develop at an early age. Suicide rates for men are higher than those of women, which may reflect men's inability to solicit help when needed.

One final thought: in the beginning of this chapter, it was stated that defining the concept of masculinity is not an easy task. It is equally difficult for me, as a man, to write about without having strong emotions. Recently, a client responded to a comment of mine regarding the rules of masculinity with this statement, "It sounds like you're pretty mad about what men have to accept, is that right? I guess we just have no choice though. It just goes with the territory." I reminded him that we are not mandated to adhere to these myths and stereotypes, especially when they have such profoundly negative consequences on ourselves and on our relationships.

REFERENCES

Balswick, J. (1979). The inexpressive male: Functional conflict and role theory as contrasting explanations. *Family Relations, 28*(3), 331–336.

Balswick, J., & Avertt, C. (1977). Differences in expressiveness, gender, interpersonal orientation, and perceived parental expressiveness as contributing factors. *Journal of Marriage and the Family, 38*(1), 121–127.

Balswick, J., & Peck, C. (1971). The inexpressive male: A tragedy of American society. *Family Coordinator, 20*(2), 363–368.

Bear, S., Berger, M., & Wright, L. (1979). Even cowboys sing the blues: Difficulties experienced by men trying to adopt nontraditional sex roles and how clinicians can be helpful to them. *Sex Roles, 5*(1), 191–198.

Carrigan, T., Connell, B., & Lee, J. (1987). Towards a new sociology of masculinity. In H. Brod (Ed.), *The making of masculinity*. Boston: Allen & Unwin.

Chodorow, N. (1978). *The reproduction of mothering*. Berkeley: University of California Press.

Chodorow, N. (1971). Being and doing: A cross-cultural examination of the socialization of males and females. In V. Gornick & B. Moran (Eds.), *Women in a sexist society*. New York: Basic Books.

Cooke, C. (1978). *The men's survival resource book: On being a man in today's world*. Minneapolis, MN: R.B. Press.

David, D., & Brannon, R. (1976). *The forty-nine percent majority: The male sex role*. Reading, MA: Addison-Wesley.

Dubbert, J. (1979). *A man's place: Masculinity in transition*. Englewood Cliffs, NJ: Prentice Hall.

Farrell, W. (1986). *Why are men the way they are?* New York: Berkeley Books.

Farrell, W. (1974). *The liberated man*. New York: Bantam.

Friedan, B. (1963). *The feminine mystique*. New York: Norton.

Goldberg, H. (1983). *The new male–female relationship*. New York: New American Library.

Goldberg, H. (1979). *The new male: From self-destruction to self-care*. New York: Morrow.

Goldberg, H. (1976). *The hazards of being male*. New York: New American Library.

Gould, R. E. (1982). Sexual functioning in relation to the changing roles of women. In K. Solomon, & N. Levy (Eds.), *Men in transition*. New York: Plenum Press.

Harrison, J. (1978). Warning: The male sex role may be dangerous to your health. *Journal of Social Issues, 34*(1), 65–86.

Hartley, R. (1959). Sex role pressures and the socialization of the male child. *Psychological Reports, 5*(3), 457–468.

Henley, N. (1977). *Body politics: Power, sex, and non-verbal communication*. Englewood Cliffs, NJ: Prentice-Hall.

Kahn, A. (1984). The power war: Male response to power loss under equality. *Psychology of Women Quarterly, 8*(3), 234–247.

Kamorovsky, M. (1976). *Dilemmas of masculinity: A study of college youth*. New York: Norton.

Kriegel, L. (1978). *The myth of American manhood*. New York: Dell.

La Haye, T. (1977). *Understanding the male temperament*. Charlotte, NC: Commission Press.

Lehne, G. (1976). Homophobia among men. In R. Brannon & D. David (Eds.), *The forty-nine percent majority: The male sex role* (pp. 66–68). Reading, MA: Addison-Wesley.

Levinson, D. (1978). *Seasons of a man's life*. New York: Knopf.

Lewis, R. (1978). Emotional intimacy among men. *Journal of Social Issues, 34*(2) 108–121.

Lipman-Blumen, J. (1984). *Gender roles and power*. Englewood Cliffs, NJ: Prentice-Hall.

Maccoby, E., & Jacklin, C. (1974). *The psychology of sex differences*. Stanford, CA: Stanford University Press.

Massengill, D., & Di Marco, N. (1979). Sex role stereotypes and requisite management characteristics—A current replication. *Sex Roles, 5*, 561–570.

Nathanson, C. A. (1977). Sex roles as variables in preventative health behavior. *Journal of Community Health, 3*(1), 142–155.

Naifeh, S., & Smith, G. (1984). *Why can't men open up? Overcoming men's fear of intimacy*. New York: Clarkson N. Potter.

Nichols, J. (1975). *Men's liberation: A new definition of masculinity*. New York: Penguin.

O'Neil, J. (1982). Gender-role conflict and strain in men's lives. In K. Solomon & N. Levy (Eds.), *Men in transition*. New York: Plenum Press.

O'Neil, J. (1981). Male sex role conflicts, sexism, and masculinity: Psychological implications for men, women, and the counseling psychologist. *Journal of Counseling Psychology, 9*(1), 61–80.

Pleck, J. (1982). Husband's paid work and family roles: Current research issues. In H. Lopata (Ed.), *Research in the interweave of social roles: Women and men: Vol. 3*. Greenwich, CT: JAI Press.

Pleck, J. (1981). *The myth of masculinity*. Cambridge, MA: MIT Press.

Pleck, J., & Lang, L. (1978). *Men's family role: It's nature and consequences*. Wellesley, MA: Wellesley College for Research on Women.

Pleck, J. (1976). The male sex role: Dysfunctions, problems, and sources of change. *Journal of Social Issues, 32*(3), 155–164.

Polk, B. (1974). Male power and the women's movement. *Journal of Applied Behavioral Science, 10*, 415–431.

Roy, M. (Ed.). (1977). *Battered women*. New York: Anchor Press.

Rubin, L. B. (1983). *Intimate strangers: Men and women together*. New York: Harper & Row.

Skovalt, T. M. (1978). Feminism and men's lives. *Counseling Psychologist, 7*(1), 3–10.

Solomon, K. (1981). The masculine gender role and its implications for the life expectancy of older men. *Journal of the American Geriatric Society, 29*(3), 297–301.

Stein, P., & Hoffman, D. (1978). Sports and male role strain. *Journal of Social Issues, 34*(2), 136–150.

Treadwell, P. (1987). Biologic influences on masculinity. In H. Brod (Ed.), *The making of masculinity*. Boston: Allen & Unwin.

U.S. Bureau of Census. (1984). *Statistical Abstracts of the United States*. p. 79.

Wagenvoard, J., & Bailey, P. (1978). *Men: A book for women*. New York: Avon.

·2·

Raised to Work

ROBERT PASICK

No one on his deathbed ever said,
I wish I'd spent more time on my business.
                                        PAUL TSONGAS

CENTRALITY OF WORK IN MEN'S LIVES

So central is work to the core of most men's identities that they are usually unaware of how much time and energy they devote to planning, performing, dreaming, and worrying about work. Like fish oblivious to the water that surrounds them, men are generally unconscious of their absorption with their jobs. Men's language is the language of work. When they are asked what they "do," they describe the nature of their jobs. Even as young boys, when asked what they want to be when they grow up, they know the question means, "what profession will you choose?"

Our clients' devotion to work is understandable. Most have been raised to consider work the most important part of their lives. Usually, their self-esteem is directly linked to their vocation and income (Sekaran, 1986). It can be inferred that a man's work also determines the degree of prestige he enjoys in the community, his access to power, and even marital eligibility. Further, for most men, their degree of job satisfaction and job security strongly impacts how well they relate to other family members. Most of our clients recognize that when they are tense and driven at work, they are much more susceptible to physical and emotional problems. This connection was supported in a 1980 *Wall Street Journal* poll of 306 chief executives nationwide, over 60% of whom believed that "personal and family sacrifices are needed to succeed . . . and almost one-quarter of the executives state that physical and mental health suffers" (Pelletier, 1985, p. 51).

The ideal of man as primary breadwinner, which was the unchallenged norm in our fathers' generation, is rapidly changing as we approach the 1990s. The combined forces of the Women's Movement and the changing nature of the U.S. economy have altered the traditional structure irrevocably. No longer is it enough for men to simply earn a solid paycheck. They are now expected to perform multiple roles, including child care, shopping, cooking, and house-cleaning—tasks that men have traditionally considered "women's work." Heightening the conflict is the social-consciousness movement of the 1970s and 1980s, which has prompted many men to question the value of the Judeo-Christian work ethic. No longer is work considered sufficiently satisfying in and of itself. Many men are asking themselves such questions as, "Is work enough?" and "Is total devotion to work hazardous to my health?"

For members of the underclass in our society, a disproportionate number of whom are minorities, there often is no direct route to participate in meaningful work. For many no career path is readily available. From 1970 through 1986, the unemployment rate for Hispanics and blacks was consistently 5%–10% higher than that for whites, from 10.4% in 1970 to 14.5% in 1986 (U.S. Bureau of the Census, 1987). These figures are not merely hollow statistics. They indicate a problem that not only affects the family's well-being, but the basic structure of our society. Unemployed men turn increasingly to drugs and crime. Because work is so central to a man's identity, a lack of job opportunities erodes his self-esteem and masculinity.

As family therapists, we see the changing expectations of men resulting in confusion and anger among many of our clients. They have been raised to regard work as their essential duty. For the entire period of development and training (during their youths), they were prepared to work hard and succeed at their jobs. Yet, when they reached the age where work is traditionally supposed to be their dominant concern, they found the old order had changed. What will replace the familiar structure is unknown. It is the stress of this dilemma that often requires therapy.

Even though they may not recognize it, the stress of their jobs has a profound effect on many men and their families. Though many men continue to find work a source of pride and satisfaction, countless others have little opportunity to be successful in meaningful jobs.

Many of the problems male clients bring to therapy are directly related to their jobs, which create chronic imbalances between work and other facets of their lives. Family therapists find the following examples of work-related problems quite typical of their practice.

A wife insists that her unenthusiastic husband join her in marital therapy. She feels hurt and angry because he seems to prefer being at the factory to home. He is indignant because he believes that by working overtime he is adequately fulfilling his role as father.

A man is referred to therapy by a doctor in a pain clinic. He is unreceptive to the suggestion that his severe back pain might be related to tension on his job as a certified public accountant (CPA). He cannot fathom taking time off to heal his back.

A male graduate student is unable to finish his dissertation. Despite winning numerous awards for his scholarship, he fears he will never gain his father's approval because he chose to pursue the humanities over medicine, a "real man's profession."

Another man has finally found in a relationship the kind of woman he has always sought. Still, he cannot resist an offer for a higher paying job in another city, though it will probably mark the end of his new relationship.

A salesman enters therapy to confront a drinking problem, yet he does not believe he can continue to be successful at work if he is unable to drink with his customers at lunch or on the golf course. For him, drinking is part of the job and, therefore, is difficult to eliminate despite its obvious danger.

A 70-year-old male owner of a small business refuses to consider retiring, though his work is physically taxing. He does not know what he would do with himself without working, since he has never developed a hobby, nor close friendships.

A man is consumed with hatred for his brother who was given control of the family business by their father.

A high-ranking executive in a large corporation does not manage to find time to attend family therapy appointments for his teenage son, who stays out late at night drinking.

A 40-year-old man hates his job as a hospital maintenance worker where he has worked for 16 years. Despite his dissatisfaction, he resists quitting his job because doing so would sacrifice good benefits, job security and a $25,000 salary. Still, the tension he experiences daily at work damages his relationship with his family.

Work pressures dominate the lives of all these men, which is not unusual. The connection between family problems and traditional male gender-role conditioning will be examined in greater depth in the following section.

WORK AND MALE SOCIALIZATION

By exploring the male socialization process, we can gain a greater appreciation of the difficulties men face in changing their work patterns. Many of the values and skills taught to young boys are far more appropriate for the workplace than for family life. Boys are expected to be competitive, autonomous, and independent. They learn at an early age that success is highly valued, and to achieve this they must be strong, persistent and self-reliant. These qualities reflect the Protestant work ethic of the late 19th century in the United States, where success in the increasingly industrialized country was predicated on one's ability to compete.

In the late 1980s, men are recognizing that these values are not compatible with family life. In an age of dual-career marriages and the Women's Movement, it is not surprising that competitiveness and independence seem to inhibit the capacity to sustain relationships. What is unexpected, however, is the increasing evidence that these values are not always effective in the workplace, either. The recent reevaluation of business in the United States (see, for example, Peters & Waterman, 1982, and Naisbitt, 1982) has prompted progressive U.S. businesses to substitute more cooperative management styles for the old, stiflingly competitive methods. According to one CEO, "The more you want people to have creative ideas and solve difficult problems, the less you can afford to manage them with terror" (McCormick & Powell, 1988, p. 47).

Even in the face of such developments, as soon as a male baby is born today, the conjecture begins as to what he will be when he grows up. Waiting for a plane, the author recently overheard several businessmen discuss a male colleague's financial manuevers. As with many male conversations, the conversation focused on work, success, failure, and competition. During a lull one man asked another about his newborn son. The recent father quickly produced some photos. His friends speculated on the future occupation of the 2-week-old boy. One remarked, "With hands like that, he's sure to be a quarterback for the Bears." Another joked, "He's got keen eyes; he's bound to be a lawyer." The fact that everyone is familiar with such scenes is one indication of the male's preoccupation with work, and also underscores men's competitive focus.

Competitiveness

The men we see in our practices were raised in an era where the competitive hierarchical structure of our society was, by and large, the unquestioned norm. These men almost unanimously report that the messages they heard as boys about manhood emphasized competition and pushing themselves to the limit. They heard such phrases as, "win at all costs," "work to the fullest of your potential," "don't be a sissy," and "don't get pushed around." Miller (1976) accurately observed that in our society a woman's identity has traditionally been based on her capacity to develop and maintain relationships, whereas a man's has centered on autonomy, competitiveness, and success.

For males in our culture, simply passing through puberty is not sufficient to enter adulthood. "To be a man" requires him to constantly prove himself in a highly structured, competitive arena. Manhood is not merely a static, developmental milestone. Rather, it is a status that must be earned repeatedly. He can "be a man" one moment, and if he fails to meet a challenge the next can just as easily lose the tenuous designation (in his own mind, if not in the opinion of others).

This competitive ethos, inculcated at a young age, is intended to prepare males for the "real world," i.e., the world of work. As clinicians we see that the view of the world as a battle ground is not conducive to a healthy family life. If a male client insists on perceiving his interactions with his family in a win–lose framework, he will have difficulty being empathetic or cooperative. The hallmarks of a successful relationship will elude him. Men tend to be excessively competitive in their familial relationships. All too often they react to simple disagreements as arguments that must be won, like a football game, rather than opportunities to learn about themselves, their spouses, and their children. After doing battle all day at work, they have difficulty relaxing at home, though they may badly want to do so. Their contentious work behavior too frequently is redirected at family members.

Rules of the Game

If a boy is to learn to be "successful" and competitive, learning the rules of the game is essential to his progress. Whereas most young girls are taught the nuances of emotional responses to better take care of relationships, most young boys are taught the subtleties of how the game is played to better their chances of winning. One need only observe children at play to recognize these common differences. Boys are often playing at some sort of sport, often with elaborate rules and almost always with winners and losers. They frequently spend as much time arguing—about who is out, who has the ball, who tagged whom, etc.—as they do actually playing the game. Girls, in contrast, tend to spend much of their play time pretending about relationships, with few guidelines and no winners and losers. They generally spend very little time debating the outcome of their play, and are more able to enjoy the play itself.

For males, learning the rules entails emphasizing the logical and rational aspects of their personalities. The rules give purpose to their game, and explain how to proceed at each juncture. Creativity and spontaneity are allowed to some degree, but only within the parameters of the rules.

It is again clear how such training prepares boys to be in control and get ahead, and could be valuable in a patriarchally structured society. This same mindset, unfortunately, also leaves our male clients unsure in their relationships, especially given the profound changes the past 20 years have introduced. The work setting may provide men an operational manual, but the home offers these men no convenient text to consult. Consequently, when men disagree with their wives, they complain that their spouses are not acting logically. "She has no reason to be upset with me," meaning he cannot understand her reaction. Aggravating the situation are the plasticity and vagueness of the new rules—in men's minds.

Keeping Score

Another distinctive characteristic of the male socialization process is the acute awareness of one's standing relative to others. This is accomplished by keeping score (Rubin, 1985). The male compulsion to keep score is evident as early as preschool, where arguments over who received a large portion are commonplace. "Tim got two pieces of candy . . . I only got one!" The pecking order is established in the grade school years by athletic success, e.g., the batting order on the little league team. Competition is also stressed in academics, through report cards and California Achievement Test (CAT) scores, which come complete with percentile rankings. In their conversations with their buddies, most boys debate who is bigger, who has seen more R-rated movies, who stays up later, and who has the most baseball cards.

As they enter early adolescence, most boys pour over box scores and league standings, evaluating their heroes as numerically as they do themselves. Later, the ranking obsession focuses on the size of anatomical parts and "how far" they "have gotten" with girls; and more dangerous tests such as how fast they can drive and how many beers they can consume in one night.

In high school and college, grade point average and class standing surface as benchmarks of success, for both women and men. An extreme example was a West Point graduate who reported that cadets were not only ranked according to academic performance but also the correctness of their attire, punctuality, and behavior during non-school hours. The rankings were public and determined the degree of privileges one was allowed.

The boyish simulations of adult achievements are put behind when the "real" task of manhood begins. For many men, their careers and incomes become the focal point of their lives, and most professions encourage men to quantify their success. Sales representatives, accountants, and lawyers in large firms are often ranked by their traditionally male bosses according to sales volume or number of billable hours, and these lists are published monthly. Factory workers depend on seniority for overtime. Even academia is structured; the number of articles published generally determines one's chances for tenure. Nor are therapists innocent, evident in discussions dominated by the amount of hours worked, papers presented, and referrals received.

The traditional male preoccupation with money is another indicator of the importance of numerical evaluations. Beyond simple necessity, money becomes the object of male aspirations. The past decade has witnessed several major Wall Street scandals resulting from extreme greed, in which the accused already had more money than one could reasonably spend in a lifetime. These incidents underscore how consuming money's appeal can be. Clinically, we find that the motivation to earn more money presents a substantial obstacle in altering the work patterns of our male clients.

A male client may claim that he is willing to do anything to improve his family life or health. Yet the suggestion that he concern himself less with his income than he has often surpasses his flexibility. In extreme cases, male clients view their portfolios and net worth as accurate representations of their self-worth. Until they are willing to reconsider these beliefs, it is unlikely any meaningful change can occur.

In addition to the overbearing requirements to compete, be autonomous, learn the rules, and quantify results, most men learn an equally restrictive list of "don'ts." They are not to share their feelings, especially those that reveal weakness and fear. Likewise, they should not become too emotionally involved with those at work. Talking openly about themselves or being soft with co-workers might cost them a promotion. No man wants to be perceived as a "wimp" at work. (For further discussion of this problem, see Chapter 5, this volume.)

INCOMPATIBILITY AT HOME

As discussed earlier, the principles men learned growing up are adaptive to most environments where men find themselves working. The same strategies that are rewarded at work, however, can fail miserably at home around family members. Worse, the skills required to be a successful husband and father have often been neglected in men's developmental lessons.

In the workplace one's "standing" is usually quite clearly understood, with the help of devices like organizational charts and civil service rankings. At home there exists no such convenient structure. Success in the home is more dependent on cooperation than competition. Many of our clients cannot leave work attitudes at the office. They cannot help competing with family members and consequently find themselves locked in protracted, bitter power struggles. The results can be especially damaging for children. When the father insists on winning in games and arguments, his offspring may develop low self-esteem and frustrated personalities.

Although some men attempt to adapt the rules of work to the home, their efforts are often met with little more success than Bull Meachum, the Navy father in *The Great Santini*, whose children resist him instead of growing closer. Similarly, in *The Sound of Music* only the addition of a kind nanny saves the children from the constrictive discipline of their widowed father.

Despite the father's attempts to establish a clear, consistent set of rules, the very nature of family life makes this a virtually impossible task. Children are not static in their development, nor do siblings have identical personalities, abilities, and needs. Change tends to come to the workplace slowly, and usually, with prior notice. The dynamics of the home environment shift constantly with little or no warning: children get sick; schools schedule reporting days; repair people need to be let in; the holidays create excitement; and childrens' feelings get hurt by friends. These uncontrollable circumstances frustrate our male clients who try to run the house with strict rules and procedures.

With the family the key to success is understanding relationships. This skill is emphasized in the typical female socialization process, which stresses empathy and the expression of feelings. In contrast, typical male socialization places more emphases on competition. Consequently, men often try to manage relationships with the techniques they find effective at work, such as logic, rationality, following rules, and finding "the answer." As appropriate as they may be at work, these approaches are generally received with scorn by family members. Further, the reluctance of men to acknowledge the feelings of others and themselves leaves them at a distinct disadvantage at home.

The father's awkward transition from the work to the family environment expresses itself in many ways. Men are taught to be autonomous, yet success at home requires cooperation and trust. They are taught to measure progress, but how does one quantify one's performance at home? Is it the number of dishes washed, diapers changed, or feelings soothed? Men rely on feedback from their supervisors to evaluate their work, but spouses or children generally do not comment on how well they are doing. To show friendliness, men learn to tease and cajole. This style of communication, however, often leads to bad feelings and arguments at home. Finally, the reinforcing power of salary sustains many men through the darker moments at work. The rewards offered a husband through fatherhood, while often gratifying, are not as easily measured as the salary or recognition received at work.

In our clinical practice we see many cases where a man cannot understand how he can be successful at work, yet so ineffective in the home that he feels like a failure. Typically, when these men enter therapy they present their wives or children as the "problem." They rarely perceive themselves as failing husbands or fathers. They cite their triumphs at work as proof of their general competence, and point to the shortcomings of their family members as the explanation for the problems at home. It is only when the therapist introduces a more systemic model of the problem—one where conflicts are viewed as interactions between family members rather than the fault of one individual—that the father is able to see his role in the dilemma.

In successful therapy the man feels sufficiently safe to reveal his feelings of inadequacy and uncertainty about his role at home. Only when this trust has been established can the man consider the possibility that his principles of career success must be modified and supplemented if he is to be equally successful as a father and husband. Under the best circumstances, the man may not only be receptive to the therapist, he will believe it is not too late to learn about nurturing and compassion. His family, in turn, may begin to understand why he tends to be so "rigid" in his family relationships. It is through the process of mutual acceptance and appreciation that families can achieve more meaningful relationships at home.

WORK-RELATED CLINICAL SYNDROMES

As previously stated, most men do not enter therapy to resolve a work-related problem. More commonly they seek therapy to reduce stress in their family or to address more general concerns such as depression, anxiety, or substance abuse. Exploration of these problems, however, frequently leads to the discovery that their work is a central issue in the family. What follows are descriptions of the most common work-related maladies for men.

Workaholism

Work is obviously not a physically addictive substance, but can be considered an addiction to a process. Wilson-Schaef and Fassel (1988) define a workaholic as someone "who has a compulsive need to work, because it provides a tangible reinforcement of self-worth not found elsewhere" (p. 1). Such people may not necessarily enjoy their work, as the task itself may have lost its meaning. Yet they prefer working to anything else in their lives. When they are not working, they do not know what to do with themselves and are consequently restless and unhappy. While laboring they may feel more pride in themselves, and have more energy and less anxiety. Like an alcoholic, however, the workaholic ultimately is disappointed in the relief provided by the "substance of choice." Though the workaholic believes working will increase happiness, more often than not it does not.

Workaholics typically have difficulty sustaining family relationships. One obvious reason is the lack of time they are able to spend at home nurturing satisfying relationships. Several recent studies have determined that "the total hours spent at work each week is the most significant predictor of family strain" (Yogman & Brazelton, 1986, p. 111).

It is clear to spouses and children of male workaholics that they value their jobs more than them. This trait is not only hurtful to the family, it is often destructive to the workaholic himself. Because he relies almost exclusively on his occupation to bolster his self-esteem, the male workaholic's mood on any given day is dependent on his supervisor's evaluation or the success of his business. It is not surprising that the male workaholic lives in a state of constant tension. He worries about work when he is away from it, and is anxious about it when he is there. Whether at home or the office, therefore, he is emotionally unavailable to his family.

When people attempt to alter their workaholic patterns, the climate of work culture in the United States becomes a crucial obstacle. In large corporations or small businesses, success almost always requires hard work and long hours. The work world often requires and reinforces the workaholic tendencies of their employees. Put simply, if a worker decides to ease up, chances for advancement are greatly diminished. In some jobs, overtime is required. Even 20 years after the virtues of the "rat race" were seriously challenged, most institutions in the United States have not significantly changed their attitude toward the balance of work and family. Maternity leave is usually quite limited, and paternity leave is all but unheard of. Even where it is available, employees seldom take advantage of it (Saltzman, 1988). Workaholics thrive in most American workplaces. Consequently, such employees unintentionally permit companies to establish norms that require excessive hours from their employees, ignoring the impact on family life.

Exacerbating the problem, workaholics are often lauded as heroes by our culture as the brightest, most productive workers. In the 1988 World Series Kirk Gibson was praised on national television by his teammates as the secret of their success because he is such a "workaholic."

Stress-Related Disorders

> "When I decided to start my business, I threw myself into it wholeheartedly. I got up at 3 every morning and would be at work by 4:30. I worked every night until 10 or 11. To build up the business I worked 7 days straight for 5 years. No days off at all. I kept up this routine until I had my heart attack shortly after my 48th birthday."

In contemporary society, where success is so highly valued, such stories are no longer shocking. That absorption with work can have a deleterious effect on physical and mental health is hardly surprising to our clients. Studies have repeatedly demonstrated the connection between work-related stress and frequent headaches, chronic back pain, ulcers, and heart disease (Pelletier, 1985). It is common to see men in therapy with stress-related disorders resulting from jobs they feel they cannot leave owing to economic or psychological reasons. These men cannot fathom making money in another field or living on less money. Other men lack the training necessary to change jobs. One client who had sold cars for 17 years was fully aware that job-related stress was the source of his chronic headaches, but he feared he could not succeed in any other field but sales. With no apparent alternatives, he felt trapped.

Some men are reluctant to relinquish high-stress jobs because of the excitement they provide. A male police officer may realize his job presents danger and anxiety, but he believes a desk job would be too boring. Some men boast about preferring a short, exciting life to a long, uneventful one. They enjoy the thrill that comes from winning (or losing) thousands of dollars in a business deal, making a tough sale, or completing a difficult computer program. Even though such behavior may be unhealthy, success and fame are revered in our culture. In *The King of Comedy*, Robert DeNiro's character Ruppert Pipkin explains his obsession with becoming a success as a stand-up comedian this way, "I'd rather be a star for a day than a shmuck for a lifetime." Such compulsions are all too common, and drive men with a force that can be frightening.

The best-known stress-related disorder is Type A behavior, which defines the behavior of "a competitive, multiphasic, achievement-oriented person who possesses a sense of time urgency and impatience, and who is both easily aroused and hostile . . ." (Wright, 1988, p. 1). Friedeman (1984) conducted numerous studies which found a significant correlation between Type A behavior and coronary heart disease.

More recent research by Wright (1988) isolated three behaviors as crucial in understanding the risk factors in Type A behavior: time urgency, chronic activation, and multiphasic behavior. "Time urgency" refers to concern over short periods of time (e.g., looking for the yellow light in order to be ready when the red changes to green). The phrase "chronic activation" refers to the tendency to stay active for most of the day, every day. Finally, "multiphasic" describes the habit of doing more than one thing at a time (e.g., reading while eating or going to the bathroom).

Wright (1988) provocatively suggests that such Type A personalities may be "hooked on their own hormones." The hormonal rush induced by their activity level may produce a chemical sensation similar to the high experienced from some drugs. Thus, some men could be dependent on their competitive nature to keep them going. To ease up would be akin to any chemical withdrawal.

Success Addiction

Success addiction is a malady similar to workaholism except that the craving is specifically for success rather than just increased time at work (Berglass, 1986). Success-addicted individuals are only momentarily satisfied with any achievement; after briefly relishing an accomplishment, they direct their career to new, more demanding goals.

Many highly successful people fit this description. They perceive most situations in their lives as "win or lose" propositions, and their careers like sporting events, complete with contests, rankings, and incentives for winning. They give little regard to their health and often have difficulty maintaining intimate relationships, in part because they treat them as competitions. These people calculate every move to determine their potential for success.

Though this syndrome is most common in men during their peak career years (25–55), it is becoming more prevalent among college-aged men and women, and even some high school students. As a sophomore in college, one male client talked to law school professors to determine what courses, experiences, and even personality traits would enhance his chances for admittance to law school. He then tailored his actions to fit this model, including the "right" classes, fraternity, offices, organizations, and summer jobs. This obsession with success became ingrained, until the success itself became the entire focus of his energy and satisfaction. Ultimately, he was unable to derive any pleasure from college life, and began to suffer from anxiety attacks and depression.

The side effects of this success syndrome can be devastating. Berglass observed, "When people focus on the outcome as opposed to the process of achieving success, one's day-to-day activities tend to lose meaning" (Cunneff, 1986, p. 97). By the time young men enter their chosen profession they are often so exhausted that they suffer burn-out before they actually begin their careers. Success addiction often leads to persistent dissatisfaction, for their goals are either unrealistic or, at best, provide only temporary fulfillment. LaBier, a psychologist who has studied this syndrome, concluded, "More and more successful people are becoming troubled, conflicted or emotionally damaged by their work and career climb. Success is a disappointment, an ending for many people" (Goleman, 1986, p. 1).

In its most extreme forms, success addiction leads to unethical or illegal actions. The Wall Street scandals of 1987 might be seen as manifestations of an obsession for success and money, one so great that it eclipsed all other concerns for themselves and their families. The potential danger of such behavior is obvious.

Work Dissatisfaction and Underemployment

Unhappiness with one's job and underemployment are more subtle but no less destructive forms of work-related stress. Work dissatisfaction is a broad-based problem with a variety of symptoms. The most common is discord with one's boss. A client described a situation where he was not getting along well with a supervisor or partner. His work history revealed a chronic problem, including numerous jobs, each one left because he could not tolerate the person in charge. He complained that the supervisor was ignorant, insensitive, and otherwise inadequate. Inevitably, this frustrated worker would return home depressed or angry, which naturally affected the entire family.

At its best, therapy can help such men explore unresolved conflicts, often with fathers, who were very domineering and critical. The adult sons may be desperately seeking from their boss approval that they never received from their father. With such foundations, it is not surprising that strained relations emerge at work.

The underemployed man believes he is performing a job that is not tapping his true potential for excellence. Such men suffer from a sense of underachievement. This feeling of failure is not always related to money or prestige. Some men who make substantial salaries are discontent because they feel the means of earning the money are below their abilities, or are not respected by their families or society. For example, one man ran the family plumbing supply business with great financial success, yet he regretted his decision not to pursue a career in journalism or academia. Our culture places a premium on the type of job a man holds. Consequently, failure to obtain a personally or socially acceptable position can be devastating. Even more traumatic for most men—and their families—is the prospect of unemployment.

WORK IN A CHANGING SOCIETY

The dramatic increase of women in the labor force over the past decade has had a tremendous impact on the male role as "breadwinner." Men are quite simply no longer the sole source of financial support for the family. From 1975 to 1987, the percentage of married mothers working rose from 44.5% to 55.8%, an increase of over 25% (U.S. Bureau of the Census, 1987). In our clinical practices we see that this change often presents increased complexity and difficulty for families. A direct result is the expectation that husbands are supposed to perform more domestic chores. If both spouses work, it is no longer clear who is responsible for the cooking, cleaning, washing, and shopping. More troublesome is taking care of the children, which is no longer the exclusive domain of the woman.

Men are faced with increased obligations, but recent research indicates that husbands in dual-career families have not significantly increased their contribution to accommodate these new roles. The ideal, where husbands and wives share evenly in the parenting and maintainance of the house, is rarely a reality. Currently, when women enter the work force they also continue to do most of the child care and housecleaning. A 1987 *New York Times* survey (Burros, 1988) found that men married to working women reported doing only 18% of the shopping and 15% of the cooking. Furthermore, the survey reports a significant discrepency between the spouses' estimations of the man's contribution. The women said the men did only 9% of the shopping and 10% of the cooking.

There are numerous reasons for men's reluctance to increase their participation. The following are the most common we see in therapy.

1. Men are ill-prepared to fill these roles. Most of our male clients simply have not been trained to cook, clean, or raise children. Not surprisingly, they do not feel confident performing these tasks, and tend to avoid them. Their insecurity is most acute in child care. Men often require considerable education to care for children of any age, especially infants.

2. Many men consider these duties "unmanly." Their socialization has taught them to regard work outside the home alone as the man's role, with child care and housecleaning disparagingly labeled "women's work." Completing these tasks on a regular basis is consequently perceived as an indication of a lack of masculinity or, worse, as evidence of a "feminine," "sissy" side. Often our clients report being chided by other men when they spend time in the kitchen or babysitting.

3. Women are not always willing to completely sacrifice these roles, perhaps due to the expectations of their own socialization. In many dual-career marriages the man may be happy to assume more responsibility for the children and home, but the woman insists on doing it herself. Couples often argue over who is the boss of the house. Sometimes, the man may be eager to do these chores, but only if he can do so independently, thus preserving a facet of his traditional male values. Likewise, the woman may want the man to share in the work, but only if she can dictate how the job is done. A power

struggle ensues over whose method is "right," which creates resentment and anger for both parties.

4. Both spouses may lack sufficient energy to fulfill the roles of employee and homemaker. As demonstrated in the earlier discussions of workaholism and success addiction, work makes tremendous demands on time and energy. "There just is not enough time to do it all," is a standard refrain of couples in therapy.

5. Employers frequently offer little or no support for men and women trying to balance the demands of work and family, and regularly require them to work past the established hours. If one wants to progress in most companies, it is necessary to work well in excess of 40 hours per week, travel regularly, and be willing to relocate.

Women at Work

The introduction of women to the workforce has also affected men on the job itself. Many men we see professionally are anxious about the addition of women at their places of work, which traditionally have been exclusively male enclaves. In professions such as sales and construction, women workers have been met with considerable resentment. Moreover, deeper conflicts result when men have women bosses, which conflicts directly with the male socialization process. Some men complain that a woman was promoted due to affirmative action, not merit. Such grievances often mask a deep sense of frustration with the difficulty of career advancement.

Another problem husbands have with women in the labor force is the loss they may feel when their own wives take outside jobs. Though men were traditionally believed to be the more autonomous sex, our experience indicates that they are very often more emotionally dependent on their spouses than women are on them. In the past, when the husband returned home after a hard day's work, the wife was there to provide emotional support, listen to his stories about work, and prepare dinner. When women work, they of course are less physically and emotionally available, and men are now expected to offer an equal amount of soothing at the end of the day. Men are occasionally confused and hurt by this change. Intellectually and economically they may support and even encourage their spouses to work, but the same time emotionally feel they may be deprived of the support their fathers' received (for further discussion of this topic, see Chapter 9).

When wives begin careers, husbands are often unsure of the appropriate reaction. The husbands may recognize the financial benefits to the family, and perhaps appreciate the potential for their spouses' growth and happiness, yet are often unable to be emotionally supportive of the move. As mentioned above, they may feel it is partly their loss, and even feel jealous that their wives are out working with other men. Furthermore, many men feel inadequate because they have not made enough money to make the change unnecessary. For many men, this is a severe blow to their sense of being "a real man."

CONCLUSION

In this chapter, we have introduced the idea that we can best understand men by first recognizing that they have traditionally been "raised to work." For generations, work has been the most important element of men's lives. However, with the addition of the Women's Movement and the changing social and economic conditions of the 1980s, "men as primary breadwinner" is a role that is rapidly evolving. Many men feel they are ill-equipped to deal with the changes. Some have become workaholics, Type A personalities, or addicted to success.

For others, the addition of women to the work force presents a common source of conflict. Husbands feel their traditional role of sole money earner is threatened, and with it their masculinity. Further complicating the situation, many men are asked to perform duties for which they are grossly ill-prepared and consider "unmanly." Even when they are willing to make such a contribution, some find their efforts thwarted by the inflexibility of their jobs or spouses. Additionally, an alarming number of men feel jeopardized by the introduction of women to the workplace, a place they assumed to be an exclusive "male enclave." Finally, these men often feel a vacuum is created by their wives going to work, which renders them less available for support at home. The recent transformation of the traditional roles have created conflicts that manifest themselves in increased familial tension.

In Chapter 7 (this volume), we will explore how to help men negotiate these vital changes. The obstacles to change will be examined, and suggestions provided to help understand and alter the patterns of work in their lives.

REFERENCES

Berglass, S. (1986). *Success syndrome.* New York: Plenum Press.

Friedeman, M. (1984). *Treating type A behavior and your heart.* New York: Knopf.

Goleman, D. (1986, August 24). The strange agony of success. *New York Times*, Section 3, p. 1.

McCormick, J., & Powell, B. (1988, April 25). Management for the 1990's. *Newsweek*, p. 47.

Miller, J. B. (1976). *Toward a new psychology of women.* Boston: Beacon Press.

Naisbitt, J. (1982). *Megatrends.* New York: Warner.

Pelletier, K. R. (1985). *Healthy people in unhealthy places.* New York: Dell.

Cunneff, T. (1986, December 8). The ladder of success may only lead to a high place to fall from. *People Magazine* p. 97.

Peters, T. & Waterman, R. (1982). *In search of excellence.* New York: . Warner Books.

Rubin, Z. (1985, November 3). Keeping score. *New York Times Magazine.*

Saltzman, A. (1988, June 20). *U.S. News and World Report*, pp. 67-70.

Sekeran, U. (1986). Self-esteem and sense of competence and moderators of the job satisfaction of professionals in dual career families. *Journal of Occupational Behavior,* 7(4), 341.

U.S. Bureau of the Census. (1987). *Statistical abstract of the United States* (108th ed.) (pp. 381, 384). Washington, DC: U.S. Department of Commerce.

Wilson-Schaef, A., & Fassel, D. (1988). *The addictive organization.* New York: Harper Religious Books.

Burros, M. (1988, February 24). Women: Out of the house but not out of the kitchen. *New York Times*, p. 1.

Wright, L. (1988). *American Psychologist, 43*(2), 1.

Yogman, M. W., & Brazelton, T. B. (Eds.). (1986). *In support of families.* Cambridge, MA: Harvard University Press.

·3·

Men as Husbands

BARRY GORDON and RICHARD METH

She looks sleek and she seems so professional
She's got a lot of confidence, it's easy to see
You want to make a move
But you feel so inferior
Cause under that exterior
Is someone who's free

BILLY JOEL, 1986

When the truth you found to be lies,
And all the joy within you dies—
Don't you want somebody to love,
Don't you need somebody to love,
Don't you love somebody to love
You'd better find somebody to love

DARBY SLICK, 1967

Harry is a 48-year-old sales representative. He's been fairly successful, which he attributes to hard work, thoroughness and care in what he does, and his ability to appear confident and knowledgable. His three grown children are all out of the house. Although he spends a great deal of time on the road he looks forward to coming home to his wife after each trip.

Lorraine, Harry's wife, recently completed a college degree she started before their first child was born. She has her first full-time job and is just beginning to feel some confidence about her teaching career. After years of feeling dependent on Harry, she has grown used to having the house to herself and managing many things on her own. However, within hours after he comes home, she hears comments from him about something she's not done at home and how busy she seems to be with her new job. Years of her pent-up anger surface. She resents being made to feel secondary to his career and jealous of his aura of competence. Harry is angry because he feels she has abandoned him. Moreover, he cannot understand her intense reaction when he believes he has been well-intentioned. Both are frustrated that his homecomings so quickly deteriorate into bitter arguments.

Harry and Lorraine represent a problem that has unfortunately become quite common in the United States over the past 20 years. The recent flood of books and media coverage criticizing men's shortcomings has not helped to defuse the tense and potentially explosive nature of male–female relationships. The Harrys of this country generally do not feel the Lorraine's accusations are true of them, and worse, they believe they are being blamed for the very things that Lorraine and their children have needed them to be. They do not know what they are supposed to be, nor what to do about it.

In this chapter we will present a picture of men in their relationships with women that we believe will be helpful in breaking the existing stalemate. Much of the division between men and women lies in their inability to understand each other and even themselves in relation to the other gender. Men and women have powerful attitudes and expectations of each other that cause them to react differently to the other gender than they do to their own gender. We will explore these expectations and attitudes, particularly from the male perspective, and seek to explain what forces have shaped them and made them difficult to change. With this understanding, we delineate the misconceptions that now exist, and lay the groundwork for men and women to overcome the tension between them.

Although much of this chapter focuses on men in their roles as mates or husbands, we should note that it may also be helpful in understanding the broader dynamics of men's relationships with women.

NEED FOR SELF-DISCOVERY: MEETING THE FROG PRINCE

In therapeutic work with couples there is an exercise that asks each member of a couple to fantasize a metaphorical representation of their spouse. Some of the common metaphors from the women in these relationships reflect the sense that their husbands are unreach-able, inflexible, and not motivated toward self-examination or change: a large rock with jagged edges, a paperweight, a statue, an oak tree, a Hitler, a Napoleon, a Henry VIII, a skunk, a bear, a lion, a dog. "You can't teach an old dog new tricks" is certainly an adage that reflects what many of these women feel about their husbands.

A woman therapist recently remarked to one of us, "Men are so damn difficult to work with. I feel like I just can't get through to them." If we as men are indeed so impenetrable, the change process clearly faces a formidable challenge.

Fairy tales often symbolize how a culture views personal transfor-mations. One popular fairy tale, "The Frog Prince," reflects many of the requirements for change by each gender.

In one version of "The Frog Prince," a beautiful young princess loses her golden ball, which the frog agrees to retrieve if the princess promises to let him play, eat, and sleep with her in return. When the princess forgets her promise, the frog follows her and demands that she keep it. The king becomes involved and insists that his daughter honor her word. After the frog agrees to sleep in her bed, the princess rebels and smashes the frog against her bedroom wall. This act breaks the spell and the frog is transformed into a handsome prince worthy of the princess.

The frog only becomes a prince when the princess defies her father and acts autonomously. Out of her strength to be herself comes the frog's chance to be liberated, but the frog must also be freed from his dependency on the princess. He has to be severely shaken up to let go of his ugly, masked self and become someone worthy of the princess' love.

Kolbenschlag (1979) uses fairy tales to illuminate the struggle by women to achieve a liberation. When it comes to men, Kolbenschlag sanguinely notes that a man rejected by a woman as a frog has a choice: "He can commit himself to an arduous pilgrimage of trans-formation . . . or he can sink into self-pity and remain fixed in his blindness. . . . He may never know that he is a frog" (p. 208).

The previous quote suggests that men are not only perceived as resistive to change; they may not even be aware of a need for change. Clearly, for any modification to occur, men must first recognize its importance, and for this to happen they may need to be shaken up. It is often a wife's threat of divorce that leads otherwise reluctant husbands to look at themselves with a critical eye. Self-awareness does not have to come only through a traumatic event. It is possible for men to achieve a better understanding of their behavior, and what has shaped it, without that knowledge being perceived as threatening or judgmental. It is this kind of self-awareness in men that we hope to foster in the pages that follow.

BEING A HERO AND ITS CONSEQUENCES

To understand why men seem to be so impenetrable, again it might be useful to examine what fairy tales tell us about how we conceive male–female relationships. Among the most well-known fairy tales that deal with feminine transformation are "Cinderella," "Snow White," and "Sleeping Beauty." Fairy tales are often much more complex than a superficial reading might reveal. These three tales depict the transformation of a fair maiden aided by the help of a princely figure. Through patience, endurance, and goodness a better life will come to these women; it is a passive evolution. The knight in shining armor, however, assumes a very active role in rescuing. It is the male's responsibility to bring happiness through his bravery. It is all but impossible to find a male protagonist in need of rescue by a woman waiting in the wings.

To become a champion of the troubled is a romantic ideal for males as soon as they are able to turn their small fists and fingers into a human gun and shoot the bad guys. This goal, however, carries an emotional price tag that defines proper male behavior. It has been part of what has traditionally been an essential aspect of male develop-ment—the differentiation of oneself from the female. From an early age, boys are set on a mission that Freud called, "the repudiation of femininity" (Monick, 1987)—a virtual obsession to demonstrate that they have no feminine traits to dilute their masculinity. As described in Chapter 2, there are powerful cultural messages that promote this attitude. Perhaps the primary manifestation of this antifemininity can be seen in the mother–son relationship. Becoming too close to one's mother, a "mama's boy," is seen to be threatening to one's "masculin-ity." Boys are expected to act as though they were autonomous, which requires considerable distance from their mothers.

Boys tend to view their mothers as resisting their independence, a perception often supported by their father's attitudes. Thus, boys may fear that their mother will consume or smother them. This concern prompts many boys to maintain an emotional distance from their mothers.

Carl Jung saw men attempting to resolve their fear of being consumed by their mothers through playing the role of "hero" (Monick, 1987). In myths and fairy tales, male heroes are indisputably masculine and, thus, the very antithesis of feminine. A male hero achieves this status by conquering a rigorous, risky challenge, far from the protection of his mother. This obstacle is frequently a lonely journey. Often, the male hero is naive and in need of help from others, but the help comes from strangers, usually not the male hero's parents, and certainly not his mother. At the end of the difficult journey his courage is verified, and the reward is usually the love of a fair maiden.

This presents an ironic element in male development. A man has not proven his masculinity until he has renounced the support of one woman and won the support of another. Paradoxically, without a woman, a man's masculinity is dubious. Gordon Cooper, one of the original "right stuff" astronauts, reflects how ancient romantic tales remain active in modern circumstances. Because his wife left him, he feared he would not be accepted into the astronaut program, which evaluated every facet of a candidate's being. He pleaded with her to return. When he became a finalist in the program she returned and he was selected as an astronaut (Farrell, 1986).

The renunciation of "femininity" is central to the development of male identity, but it is not without negative consequences. One of the legacies of this process is an "unfinished sense of vulnerability and loneliness" (Osherson, 1986, p. 105) from childhood. Psychoanalytic theory tells us that, as part of female development, girls must learn to relinquish attachment to their fathers and are encouraged to strengthen their bond with their mothers. Boys normally follow a reversed pattern, but the parent with whom they are to identify has been the traditionally absent, inaccessible father. Boys, then, do not simply sacrifice mother's nurturing; later they give up nurturing altogether, which results in vulnerability and loneliness.

RELATIONSHIPS WITH WOMEN

Males, then, enter their adult quest for female companionship with an emptiness to fill. They not only need to prove themselves to a woman and their peers, but also have a deep unconscious desire for the nurturing from which they sloughed off at an early age. Rubin (1983) asked a man who had recently become a father what his marriage meant to him. "I had been lonely for a long time—a long time. Then when I got married, it changed. I finally had someone in my life who was really there for me . . . it was like coming home again" (p. 61).

In the metaphor exercise for couples mentioned earlier, the most common representations by husbands of their wives were mother figures. It was also quite common, however, for the husbands to depict their wives as objects or pets (such as plants, flowers, bunnies, or dogs) that needed to be taken care of. These two opposing images—the caretaker and the object to be taken care of—reflect an inherent conflict central in men. Men want to be dominant protectors, but they also want mothering. This can result in a fear of intimacy lest they be smothered. It was telling that the husbands were usually posing as observers in their metaphorical descriptions. They may have felt closeness and involvement, but they remained at a distance.

The caretaker and protector roles have also been addressed by Scarf (1987), who identified one common type of unconscious marital contract which puts one partner in the role of the fragile person (usually the wife), the "wounded bird," and the other as caretaker (usually the husband), presumably to care for this frail bird. A different version of this arrangement results when a woman uses marriage as a means of leaving her home of origin. In this paradigm, the husband becomes *in loco parentis*, the provider of home and security, even though he may also be leaving his home of origin for the first time. With the present generation of career-minded women working outside the home, these dependent arrangements are perhaps less common or less pronounced than in the past, but emotional dependence has certainly not vanished between the genders, and can occur in either direction.

Men enter relationships expecting to be dominant, and take care of the "weaker sex." After all, a man does not win a maiden through heroism only to relinquish the rewards and responsibilities. Men may readily accept this role, yet unconsciously desire something different. Still, they generally behave in ways that discourage a balanced relationship. As a result, they continue to carry within them a longing to be nurtured and to have someone *they* can depend on.

When women accept a dependent role, it becomes that much more difficult for men to transcend their "masculine" roles. Men may resent the burdens and limitations of their roles, and may react out of that resentment in the manner that women criticize, i.e., being insensitive, unapproachable, or even hostile. There are a myriad of factors that must be considered to understand why men tend to resist changing a role pattern that they do not like.

MALE EXPECTATION TRAP

To understand how men become entrapped in structures that restrict their behavior and expression, it is useful to examine expectations that women commonly have of men, that men have of themselves in relating with women, and that our culture prescribes for men in interactions with women. These expectations outline which duties each gender fulfills and the stereotypes we develop.

Farrell (1986) perceptively remarked that both sexes often see themselves as powerless in exactly the areas in which the other believes they are powerful. Conversely, one partner tends to see strength in the other where he or she feels weak. Men, for example, tend to see women as adept at handling children, relationships, social situations, domestic responsibilities, and emotions. Women generally see men as competent with money, business relationships, and mechanical operations.

It is not only men who believe it is their responsibility to be successful economic providers; women also continue to expect men to perform those tasks, believing that men know more about such matters. The result is a reinforcement of the model where men are good providers for their families if they are oriented to success in the economic world.

The dramatic shift in the number of women working has not substantially altered these expectations, despite the decline of womens' economic dependence on men. Farrell (1986) found that the more money the husband makes, the less likely it is that his wife works. This finding might suggest that men prefer women to remain financially dependent on them. But if many women choose not to work when given the opportunity, this reinforces men's beliefs that there is a strong connection between their economic success and their desirability to a woman.

Money is only one of the conventional gender-based expectations that surface in relationships. Women still often expect men to handle mechanical problems and take care of the yard. Men, of course, have their own expectations of women, including that they will do the cooking, cleaning, and laundry. Both spouses' expectations are based more on custom than gender imperatives. Men are no more biologically equipped to mow the lawn than women are to tuck the kids in at night; yet, it's what many believe they are expected to do. Most men refuse to challenge these stereotypes for fear of appearing "unmanly."

At a workshop given by us, one man expressed his dilemma this way: "When I am expected to show my strength to a woman, that is actually when I feel most vulnerable. When I can be vulnerable and let out my feelings, that is when I feel strong with others." When women convey expectations that men perform their traditional duties, they may unknowingly reinforce men to occupy roles that are familiar but which block men from expressing their "softer" side, something many women want from men. Maintaining these prescribed roles satisfies some of the ego and security needs of each gender. However, they not only originate from these needs, they are also a response to expectations that have deeply entrenched cultural roots. Both genders are exposed to similar messages that socialize them to expect gender-based behaviors.

One of us called an answering service and was greeted by a laughing operator. The operator explained that "The Newlywed Game" was on, and one contestant was asked, "What is overdeveloped and what is underdeveloped about your husband?" The young wife answered, "My husband has an overdeveloped ego and an underdeveloped checkbook!" It may not have been a coincidence that ego and checkbook went together. For too many men and women, the state of development of a man's ego depends on the balance in his checkbook. Perhaps a more perceptive woman might have seen her husband as having an overdeveloped focus on his checkbook as a way of compensating for an underdeveloped ego.

The electronic media reinforce the traditional male image by offering few role models to compete with the popular images of "strong," emotionally repressed, handsome men. Unfortunately, when men are not portrayed as tough, macho heroes, they are more likely to be wimpy buffoons than men who are expressive in a way that reflects depth of character. Farrell (1986) argued that men in the media appeal to women because of their strength and success, rather than sensitivity and caring. The media suggest that a man should be wealthy enough to buy what his woman wishes. These are the values that many of us grew up with, and they still shape our beliefs about manhood. The insidious nature of these influences makes it impossible to separate what men should be for themselves from what women want them to be. Men are conditioned, in part, to aspire to be what women supposedly want them to be, while women are conditioned to believe men should appeal to them in this way.

THE BURDEN OF MALE STRENGTH

Many men are taught to believe that masculinity is validated more by strength than any other quality, and that this has great appeal for women. "Strength" can be demonstrated in many ways, including self-sufficiency, invulnerability (not showing physical or emotional weakness), and tenacity (completing what is asked of you no matter what it takes). Monick (1987) concludes that the fundamental mark of maleness, the phallos, represents "sinew, determination, effectuality, penetration, straightforwardness, hardness, strength." Men believe they should be able to perform sexually or materially, without help and regardless of their emotions or circumstances. A line from *Zorba the Greek* (Kazantzakis, 1952) typifies this attitude. Zorba is a free-spirited "man's man," who tries to develop a timid friend's masculinity: "If a woman sleeps all alone, it's the fault of us men . . . God will forgive all sins . . . But that sin he will not forgive" (p. 106).

Part of being a male, then, is to persistently come through. Some men are haunted by any failure or sign of weakness, and hence attempt to maintain an aura of impenetrability and invulnerability. A friend's father returned from World War II with part of his leg blown away. This friend could not recall any conversation between his parents about this crippling condition until his father fell going up some steps. The mother instinctively reached out to help her husband, only to be greeted by a tirade. To have his limitation exposed by an offer of help was more than this man could bear.

A colleague's car recently caught fire in their driveway and, despite the obvious danger of an explosion, her husband raced for a fire extinguisher from the kitchen and tried to put out the fire himself. His wife, on the other hand, immediately called the fire department.

This husband acknowledged his wife's good sense, and was personally alarmed at how instinctively he tried to resolve this situation alone, placing himself at tremendous risk.

Men are commonly criticized for not expressing emotions. Part of the conditioning men receive from the time they are little, as we have noted elsewhere, is to conceal emotions, especially those indicating "weakness," such as fear and sadness. Men are not raised to be insensitive, they are raised to keep going regardless of their feelings. The message is, "Don't be overcome by your feelings," not, "Don't show any feelings at all." However, it is much easier to block feelings altogether than to release measured amounts and hope that you are not overcome in the process. Men who do not express feelings are not necessarily rejecting feelings per se, but are protecting their masculine image.

To remain seemingly invulnerable, men must not only be able to surmount their feelings, but must also not allow themselves to express needs. Needs, after all, inherently leave one vulnerable. Because they feel they must deny their needs, men become victims by their need to deny vulnerability. Like the crippled man who fell, men tend to act as though they can bear anything, and do without everything. Again, as with feelings, it is not that men have no needs, but that revealing them contradicts the image men believe they must present. Denying needs is a way, then, to protect one from feeling vulnerable.

Men can often be so adept at their denial that they may not even be conscious of their needs. A wife in marital therapy ignored her husband's usual disclaimers and bought him some new underwear. Over such a mundane purchase, the husband had tears in his eyes. He explained that no one ever gave him anything, though of course he always discouraged people from doing so. His strong reaction shocked him and revealed that, though he could not admit it, he had hoped someone would think of him. In the past he might have gotten angry at his wife for the purchase, yet he would also have accumulated resentment for all the times his needs were overlooked. The years of self-denial had caught up with this man, and he could no longer be a "good" male martyr.

The male pattern of self-denial is one that can be traced, at least in part, to the early messages from fathers and society, which tell boys to not seek too much affection, in general, even from their mothers. A boy who accepts too much maternal attentiveness is regarded as a "mama's boy." The theory is that a boy "tied to his mother's apron strings" will allow himself to be smothered by his mother's nurturing and will then be too "soft" and unfit to meet the harsh demands of the world with self-sufficiency and endurance. Boys learn to avoid this risk by acting as though they have no need whatsoever for any affection, a belief instilled by our society.

DENIAL AND DEPENDENCY

The male code of self-denial also means not expecting to have one's needs met. However, men can generally allow themselves some attentiveness without feeling unmanly. Despite their unwillingness or inability to voice most of their significant needs, men commonly define some needs they consider acceptable. They use this list to measure attentiveness by their female mates. For some husbands this means having dinner on the table, the house clean, or their wives dressed up when they return. Many men will react with strong, even irrational anger to such "slights" or "disrespect for my simple wishes" if these expectations are not met. Underlying this anger is a feeling of abandonment. Few men make this emotional connection directly because they are not in touch with their more fundamental needs.

Osherson, in *Finding Our Fathers* (1986), admits "perhaps in our need to defend and constantly protect women we are trying to tiptoe past the rage we feel if they leave us too much alone" (p. 123). Such unexplained rage may compel women to keep a safe distance. However, this may feed men's sense of abandonment. It may also lead some women to fear not meeting these camouflaged needs for attentiveness. So, ironically, women and men play out a charade that keeps both partners from acknowledging what each really needs and feels.

There are some times when men do reveal their needs in more direct ways. However, some women react with alarm to the neediness expressed by their partners (Scarf, 1987). This may be due in part to their unfamiliarity with such male vulnerability or their discomfort with the introduction of new emotional demands. Again, the outcome will likely be a shift back to traditional, expected behavior. Many husbands in therapy indicate that they have attempted to respond to their wives' requests for more expression, but felt that these efforts were ignored and withdrew in frustration.

Although many of men's denied needs are material, some are clearly emotional. One form of deprivation many men inflict on themselves is a lack of supportive, intimate connections. A full chapter in this book is devoted to the issue of how men deal with friendships, but it is not only the men who are affected. Their female partners also suffer as a result of their asceticism. Men in therapy, with inordinately high frequency, acknowledge that not only are their wives or girlfriends their best friends, but their only truly close friends, the only people they feel free to confide in. Often these men will have one or a few close "buddies," but will not share any important conversations with these friends.

The concentration of his emotional needs in one relationship, with his wife, creates a strong dependence in a husband. If that one person is unavailable, the husband is prone to feel alone and hurt. This is often the underlying cause of the seemingly inexplicable overreactions that women suffer when they have not met a relatively minor expectation of their husbands.

A couple in therapy had planned a trip to Europe. When the wife tried to explain her desire to leave on a return flight a few hours earlier than her husband to be back for a special social event, he became enraged and acted as though the whole trip would be spoiled. Without his best and only friend he would have felt too alone. However, his explanation for his anger was her lack of consideration for the people with whom they were travelling, not his own emotional needs.

DIVISION OF LABOR AND
ITS EMOTIONAL UNDERPINNINGS

Male dependence on women can also manifest itself in the division of domestic responsibilities. A husband's reluctance to share fully in chores is generally taken to be another facet of the inflexible macho persona. However, it may well reflect the hidden need to be dependent, to lean on someone else, and to be relieved of some of the intense sense of responsibility men commonly carry within. It is easier for a man to believe his own hard labor allows him to sit back and take it easy than to openly ask to be taken care of. Such a request would reveal the underlying vulnerability and fear of not being able to do it all, something men view as an important measure of masculinity.

We have seen a number of men in therapy who performed functions that were counter to gender stereotypes. Yet, these men were often inexplicably resistant to certain kinds of responsibility. One man who headed a department at a university said, "I deal with problems and pressure and conflict all day long. When I come home I just want things to be easy. So, when Jan brought family problems to my attention that needed to be talked about, I didn't want to hear it and the more she pushed, the angrier I got and the more I withdrew."

Another young man who had always helped with cooking and cleaning was strangely uninvolved with his newborn daughter. His explanation, when he became able to express it, was that he did not feel ready to be a father yet, nor was he ready to share his wife's attention and affection with the baby. He could even voice his anger at the baby he so obviously loved and realize that he was struggling with the fact that it was time to relinquish some of his dependent needs.

Bell, in *Being a Man* (1982), states that the struggle to maintain equality in a marriage through assigned roles often represents a deeper struggle to get one's own needs satisfied. Even in relationships that appear "equal," Bell perceptively observed that one frequently finds a continued dependence by the man on the woman. Many husbands who are fully supportive of their wives' independence still want and often expect to be taken care of. These husbands are supportive of their wives' achievements, but are not prepared to lose the nurturing they want and have come to expect.

One husband who prided himself on his independence was the sole manager of a substantial business; yet he would never schedule his own appointments for therapy. He relied on his wife, who also worked full-time, to keep their calendar. This is one of the myriad ways the division of tasks can be manipulated to secure caretaking from the other person. Conflicts between men and women over division of labor may actually be about caretaking: the desire to be taken care of in expected ways, or to assume familiar caretaking roles.

Women are generally perceived as givers, i.e., those who nurture within relationships (Gilligan, 1982). The perception is that men also give, but not "nurturing" as much as material and emotional security. They are supposed to be problem solvers. Some women may be unfulfilled by men because women, as "givers," may not present clearly their needs for nurturing. Men, however, may often not get needs met because they deny even having them. The struggle over sharing responsibilities, then, is frequently heightened because of the frustration of not having these submerged needs met.

Men today are caught between the old and the new, between holding onto the breadwinner role and trying to share more (Bell, 1982). The "old" values husbands learned from their fathers and the "new" ones introduced by their wives and the socioeconomic changes in family life are frequently not in concert.

Adult men who now help raise families are in a position to set the pattern for future generations. They are also a generation in transition. Their fathers were generally uninvolved at home. Whatever conflicts their parents experienced over sharing responsibilities or expressing feelings were typically not prevalent nor readily identifiable.

The result is a paradox: To be the kind of man women are saying they want today runs counter to the kind of men their fathers "taught" them to be. Since fathers effectively define for boys what masculinity is, many men feel that they are being asked to be someone whom their fathers would not respect. Much of this, of course, is not consciously realized; yet, such considerations are central to the psychological development of adult males and, thus, to their identities. To change according to the wishes of the present generation of adult women can be tantamount "to murdering his own self-image" (Kolbenschlag, 1979, p. 208).

Recognizing this dilemma helps us understand why such changes do not come readily. It also allows us to see how different perspectives lead to much misunderstanding. In the section that follows, we will examine how this misunderstanding effects the way men and women struggle to make their relationships work.

Success is very important to men, whether it be in the workplace, athletic field, or home. If you ask men to reflect on whether they live up to what's expected of them as husbands, most will say they are responsible and provide well. Yet many will also admit that the feeling of success they enjoy at work eludes them as husbands. We present a number of vignettes that poignantly reveal the conflicts men feel as husbands. Some are excerpts from clinical interviews.

To assure greater balance, we interviewed men of different ethnic and socioeconomic backgrounds. These were not clinical interviews with current or past clients; these were interviews with men willing to participate strictly on a voluntary basis. We placed an ad in the university newspaper asking for male volunteers to discuss their lives in confidence with a faculty member doing research on the subject.

Because we wanted to learn about men who had experienced being a husband and father, we specifically asked for married men, between the ages of 25 and 65. These interviews unearthed an assortment of painful feelings that the men had obviously tried to bury or ignore.

BEING A HUSBAND: JOHN'S STRUGGLE

John, 45 years old and married to the same woman for 23 years, seemed eager to discuss the subject of being a husband. I asked him to relate to me the kind of husband he feels he is, from his and his wife's perspective:

> JOHN: Believe it or not, it's something I'm never quite sure of. . . . I think I do OK, but I never really know whether Betsy appreciates what I do or if what I'm doing is enough. I do well in my job, and bring home a pretty good chunk of money, but if you ask Betsy about it, she'll tell you she doesn't care about the money, which I doubt, by the way.

> INTERVIEWER: What does she want from you?

> JOHN: That's the problem; I don't know. Except for talking with her; yeah, that is something she always complains about. I don't talk about things the way she does. You know how women are, they want to hear about how you feel about this and that, but there's just so much of that kind of talk I can do. Even when I do talk with her about what I feel or think, she tells me I'm not letting her know what's really inside of me. It's frustrating, because no matter what I do, it's not enough. It's like I hear more about what I don't do than what I do.

> INTERVIEWER: Do you think you are really telling her what's inside you?

> JOHN: Well, I don't know, I've always been a pretty private person. Maybe not as much as I should.

For many men, being "a private person" euphemistically expresses one of the cardinal rules men subscribe to: Pay little heed to your feeings or, better, deny them altogether. At the least, keep them to yourself. There are few qualifiers to this rule; most wives are not privy to all their husbands' private thoughts. Men learn to not discuss feelings since this will reveal vulnerability, weakness, and suggest a more "feminine" orientation. So what happens when John is troubled about something? Does John deliberately avoid talking with Betsy? The problem for Betsy is that John may not even know he has a problem. I asked John about this:

> JOHN: It's a funny thing, and something Betsy cannot understand. Some things either just don't bother me, or I work them out myself without realizing it. I've never been the kind of person to talk about my problems with anyone. Somehow they get worked out, because I don't talk about them, not with Betsy or with my friends.
>
> INTERVIEWER: When you were a kid, did you talk with anyone about personal things? What about your parents?
>
> JOHN: No, not really, especially with my dad. Actually, I do remember one time when I was 16 and had a problem with this guy I worked for on my summer job. One day this guy did something which got me really upset. That night I told my old man about it and his reaction was basically to accept it, that it's going to happen at any job, you just have to learn to live with it. He also went on to tell me that there were things about his job he didn't like, but if he complained about those things he never would have moved up in the company. Nobody likes a bellyacher, he used to say. Plus, I look at how emotional Betsy gets about the smallest things. It's something I couldn't deal with, that's for sure. It's especially hard when I take it [his emotions] to work. Like my old man said, nobody likes a complainer.

John sensed both his need to be in control and his preoccupation with handling matters alone. With messages like "don't bellyache," John has been conditioned to internalize and deny feelings. This is the male creed. With his wife, however, this habit is problematic. As Betsy's husband, John hears other messages and is exposed to different expectations. Betsy wants him to talk about himself, his day, and his struggles. It is unthinkable to Betsy that John would not need to come home and use her as a sounding board. John has needs, so to her this makes perfect sense. But John does not focus on his emotional needs.

John may not realize his wife's expectations conflict with his and other's expectations of how he should feel and act. What he is aware of, however, is the discomfort he feels at home, a place where he feels confused and unhappy. It took John and Betsy some time to understand this conflict, and, as with many couples, only after many years of struggling with their relationship. John described it this way:

JOHN: One of Betsy's other main gripes is that I spend too much time at the place [workplace]. I hate to admit it, but she's right.

INTERVIEWER: Do you need to be there as much as you are?

JOHN: No, not really (John pauses, looks down at the ground, and then looks back at me)—to be honest, I think I'm deliberately avoiding going home. It's not that I don't love Betsy and the kids; that's not it at all. But for a while there, we couldn't talk with one another without arguing. Then we're angry.

INTERVIEWER: Both of you?

JOHN: Well, not really. I would withdraw; I know that by now. I would wrap myself inside of a cocoon . . . Betsy would say I retreated into my shell. Then I would go off and think all kinds of things, like maybe I never should have married Betsy or maybe I never should have married, period. Recently, I came to the realization that I'm probably better off when I do work longer hours. At least at work I'm appreciated; my performance there is usually in the top 5%. I don't make waves there; I just do my job without bellyaching. My boss, the V.P., they're all pleased with my work . . . (long pause) . . . It's good there.

INTERVIEWER: (Here it appeared that John was running out of steam) It sounds like you feel fairly successful at work, that you do a pretty good job. But it doesn't sound like you feel very successful with Betsy. Is my impression correct?

JOHN: You're right . . . (he pauses) . . . I don't feel good there, and that's crazy, since a man should feel good in his own house. But I don't.

John's frustration mirrors his wife's, and represents the struggle of many men who try unsuccessfully to fulfill their responsibilities as husbands. Throughout marriage, John has struggled with the word "husband." What were his expectations? Was he prepared to take on the responsibilities this role carries? Why does he feel so unappreciated when he works so hard to be a caring and loving husband?

Like many men, John has been oblivious to the mostly covert, powerful influences that gender-role conditioning has had on his marital relationship. Like most men, John longs to wear the ultimate badge—the badge of success. On his job, bringing in the most money is the bottom line, and he is proud that he has reached the top of his division through hard work and effort. But as a husband, he has felt like a failure. During our interview it was painfully evident that John had no idea why things had not worked out the way he had hoped with

Betsy. When I asked him what had happened, he attributed the problems to things other than the influence of the male gender role. I then asked him to talk about how prepared he feels he was to take on the responsibilities as a husband. What were his initial expectations?

JOHN: I guess I was naive like most guys. I put a lot of emphasis on sex, figuring that was an important area to be compatible. Before we were married there were some problems around sex, but we worked them out, at least for awhile. Betsy was not the first woman I had a relationship with, but I kind of knew she was the one I'd end up with. We had the same ideas, same dreams about the future. She wasn't pushy, which I liked. Actually, she was pretty quiet, not at all demanding. That's definitely one thing which has changed over the years. Anyway, we talked about kids, and seemed to have the same ideas about how many we wanted, how to raise them, etc. When the kids were small it was very busy; I was busting my ass to make enough to buy us a decent home and Betsy had her hands full with the girls. We didn't really plan to have the three so close together, but it happened and Betsy seemed to handle it OK. Then I got an important promotion to district manager which helped financially. Am I answering your question?

INTERVIEWER: Yes, this is on the right track. Could you elaborate on what you said about Betsy becoming more demanding? How did that affect things?

JOHN: Oh, I think that had a pretty negative effect on our relationship, and I wasn't ready for it . . . but to be honest, I was always too domineering, at least in the beginning of our relationship. Basically, I'm a fairly opinionated person, and stubborn, so I don't like it when someone disagrees with me. Betsy finally got fed up with this; she told me I never listened to her ideas but tried to get her to accept mine. She began to complain about my not being around. I know she resented my job, although she never said that in so many words. She was right—I was away a lot—and for a while I couldn't figure it out. I didn't want to admit that I was avoiding her, but I was. I even started losing interest in sex. It was like a role reversal—instead of my pursuing Betsy, she was the one who pursued me. I became totally obsessed with work. Finally, Betsy told me she had contacted a marriage counselor. At first I thought, "No way am I going to talk to some stranger about our problems." After I calmed down I agreed to go, figuring we were not working things out on our own.

INTERVIEWER: How did that work out for you?

JOHN: It was a good move, probably saved our marriage. It's far from perfect now, but definitely better than it was.

Although I indicated that he was under no obligation to talk about his therapy, John wanted to talk more so "other guys in the same boat as me might learn something from my mistakes." In the 3 hours we spent together, more revelations came to John. It had never occurred to him that his male gender conditioning was in part responsible for not knowing anything about emotional intimacy. When I suggested that his difficulties with Betsy might have been related to what he had been taught about "manhood," John seemed amused and then struck by this notion. This discovery John received with mixed feelings:

> "Somehow I never realized this before—maybe I didn't want to ac-knowledge it—but now I can say that my success at work has been at my family's expense, especially Betsy's. But you're right; Betsy does things so much differently from me. I never talked with the guys about things the way Betsy talks with her girl friends, and that's how I think she wants it to be between us. Since we did that counseling I know I talk more about what I feel, but, still, not that much. It's upsetting, and it takes me days to recover from one of our heart-to-heart talks. Not to mention that I then have to put it out of my mind so I can function at work. Sometimes I wonder if it's worth it."

RESTRICTIONS OF THE MASCULINE MODEL

John's struggle is not unique. Becoming a husband presents some of the most conflicting feelings that men experience. To succeed as a husband means more than providing food and shelter, but many men consider these their primary functions. It also requires being emo-tionally open and sensitive with one's partner. But for a man to do this is antithetical to his conditioning. Current models of masculinity, based mostly on traditional gender roles, interfere with fulfilling basic needs of intimacy.

In order for this behavior to improve, messages to men about self-disclosure, emotional expression, and vulnerability have to change. When a man insulates himself from his feelings he distances the person with whom he chooses to have an intimate relationship. Without realizing it, he may erroneously equate attachment with dependency and weakness. The benefits of an intimate attachment are sacrificed in order to maintain a strong identification as a male.

Chodorow (1982) theorizes that due to their experience with separation and attachment in early childhood, men are ambivalent when it comes to maintaining a meaningful attachment to another individual. Perhaps for this reason, men are viewed as the distancer in relationships (Rubin, 1983). Although sweeping generalizations like this can be unfair, there is some justification to this.

There are a variety of ways that men can be intimate and give emotionally. How does a man connect to the person with whom he wishes to share in a permanent, monogomous relationship? With feelings of attachment for this special person, men may also have numerous expectations for their physical, sexual, and emotional needs being satisfied. What most men do not realize is that for everything they hope and wish for there are contradictory demands to remain loyal to all they have internalized about being male. Our current models of masculinity present men with a conflictual dilemma. A man who plays by the rules will be totally invested in his work and feel this is sufficient. The man who does not adhere to traditional guidelines may be more invested at home, more available to his wife and children, but feel inadequate before other men. And like John, many men might find they are unhappy but cannot understand or articulate what is happening to create this unhappiness.

All human beings need to be cared for, nurtured, and loved, yet men are not given permission by our society to pursue these basic human needs. As we noted earlier, for a man to acknowledge this fact suggests a vulnerability—a lack of strength that causes him to seriously question his sense of manhood. Boys often grow up emotionally detached and isolated from what they feel. Men unknowingly build inpenetrable walls that insulate them from the wide range of affects human beings experience. These are powerful unconscious processes that will not necessarily change because of marriage and the responsibilities that go with it.

So what do men do with the emotions that brew inside of them? If men are taught to suppress or ignore their feelings, how do they satisfy their basic human needs? The obvious answer is that many men do not. For the men who do, they find subtle, more covert ways to meet their desires. Generally, the physical or sexual dimensions of a relationship are acceptable means of expressing feelings and being nurtured. But as we will see later, even the sexual relationship provides limited fulfillment.

MALE SEXUALITY AND ITS ROLE IN MARRIAGE

When a man loves and commits to a woman, he finds ways to get closer that are comfortable and familiar to him, usually through the physical aspects of a relationship. Sexual intimacy is sometimes the sole means of how males express their affection for their partner, providing an acceptable means of emotional bonding. According to existing models of masculinity, a husband is allowed to depend on his wife for this. But for couples, sexuality can be the source of many marital battles. In our clinical practice we hear women express frustration over what they consider their husband's preoccupation with sex. Sexual intimacy may meet a man's needs but can simultaneously negate the woman's needs, who has other ways of expressing and receiving love. This is one of the more common problems marital therapists face. Irreconcilable differences and marital dissolution are not unusual outcomes.

A good example of this is Nancy, a 43-year-old part-time computer programmer, and Gene, a 44-year-old high school principal; they have two children. Gene and Nancy have been married for 19 years. Nancy, calling to make the appointment, noted that she "had one foot out the door but was giving the marriage one last chance because Gene had asked for it." When they came in, both appeared quite anxious and tense. After exchanging some pleasantries to increase their comfort, I asked each of them to tell me what had brought them to me now. Nancy wasted no time listing the areas of their relationship that were problematic for them, including their different sexual needs. The following is an excerpt of this discussion. The therapist has just asked Nancy to elaborate on the sexual problem:

NANCY: I guess I've been turned off to sex for a long time; that's all Gene ever seemed to want from me. It got to the point that I didn't even want to hug him because he thinks as soon as you touch him you want to go to bed. Even when I'm in the kitchen cooking he'd come over and touch me in a way which tells me he wants sex. So I've stopped touching him, stopped being affectionate, which has been very hard for me. It may sound ridiculous to you, but it's the truth. (pause) I've often wondered if sex is the only reason why Gene wanted to stay married to me.

GENE: Oh, come on Nancy, that's crazy and you know it. You make it sound like I'm some sex maniac or something. I like to be affectionate, too, not just for sex; the problem is that you only see things one way, so . . . (Nancy interrupts).

NANCY: Gene, let's be honest here; otherwise it's not going to help. Are there ever times you want to sit and just be together? No, and you know it. (Turning to the therapist) These problems go back a long time; ever since our kids were small. Gene doesn't work long hours and makes a good living; I have no complaints. But for him to come home and spend time with me—well, as long as he knew there was sex, he'd be happy.

GENE: Look, she makes it seem like there's something wrong when a guy wants sex. Isn't it something people do when they're married? Our sex life was great, at least until she decided she wanted to punish me by saying no all the time. Without sex there's no reason to be married. But, I don't want to be with anybody else either. (Long pause) She knows I love her, and sex is the way I show my love. It's special; that's all. She just doesn't understand that it isn't just the sex.

THERAPIST: There seems to be more, Gene. . . . What does Nancy need to know about it so she could better understand you, so she can believe that you are not just, as you say, a sex maniac?

GENE: (Hesitating, and looking a bit irritated) I don't know what to say . . . (sounding hopeless) . . . no matter what I say she has her mind made up. Maybe this counseling is a waste of time.

THERAPIST: Wait a moment. You and I both know how important it is for Nancy to understand that sex is more than just physical pleasure for you. From what you say, I get a sense that something else happens for you when you are sexually intimate with Nancy. What happens, why is that such a special time?

GENE: There's a lot of pressure at school so the one time that I can relax and feel close to Nancy is when we have sex. She knows I'm not a very affectionate person; I have never been this way. Nobody in my family was ever touchy the way they were in her family. But I'm affectionate when we're having sex. Just ask her; I'm pretty caring, not just out for myself. I guess I can express myself better when we're making love. (A long pause) It's when I really enjoy Nancy. It's not that I don't enjoy her at other times; it's just different; I feel closer I guess. I don't know if this is making any sense.

THERAPIST: It's beginning to make sense. I hear you saying that sex is the time, maybe the only time, you truly feel an emotional bond to Nancy, a special kind of closeness that somehow you don't feel at other times, is that right?

GENE: Yeah, I guess I never thought of it that way, but you're right. (He looks away, somewhat embarrassed) I feel closer to Nancy then more than any other time; I thought she knew that. Dammit, I love Nancy; why the hell is that so hard for her to realize?

THERAPIST: Maybe it's hard for her to know only by your actions. It sounds like the words you just spoke may begin to help her understand that sex is for you a means of expressing a lot of the feelings you have for her.

NANCY: (Looking a bit teary) You know, Gene has never said anything like this before, at least not to me. I had no idea he felt this way. (She turns to Gene, now steadily crying) How come with all of the arguments we've had about this, you never said this? It really would have helped.

GENE: I don't know, probably because I never realized this before we started talking today. It was when he said something about how I feel close to you that it hit me. I'm not a talker—you know that—and that is probably one of our big problems. This is something I could never put into words before tonight.

THERAPIST: No doubt that has always been a problem for you, not only with Nancy but perhaps also with others. And what ends up happening is that your behavior can often be misinterpreted, as it has by Nancy. You see, it's easy to make assumptions about behavior. But you are like many men, a man more of action and not as many words. But just now, Nancy seems to have really responded to your words. Words can be very important between a husband and wife.

NANCY: You know, sometimes I wonder whether we're speaking the same language, Gene and I. You would think that a high school principal would be able to communicate with words, since he does it all the time at work.

THERAPIST: I'm sure at work he can find the appropriate words, but when it comes to the marital relationship, it's a whole different matter. This idea about speaking two different languages is not a far-fetched idea at all. In fact, it is probably one of the underlying causes for the problems you and Gene have had with one another.

Because he grew up without mastering a language of emotional expression, Gene has only his behavior to convey his feelings. As he fumbles around for the right words, Gene feels frustration, anger, and hopelessness. He knows what he feels but struggles to convey in words the meaning of his behavior. It is important for Gene to understand that what he learned about masculinity makes it difficult to verbalize what he feels, since past models of masculinity have not allowed for this. For many men, sexual contact is where emotional intimacy happens. As Gene indicated, sex is more than physical pleasure; it's a special time. Nancy did not realize all that it meant to him, and when they attempted to discuss the subject of sex, angry and hurt feelings divided them even further.

Words about feelings are rarely accessible to men, and therapists need to help couples understand this. When a couple learns that there is probably nothing deliberate or malicious about a man's interest in sex—that it may be the man's only known means of connecting emotionally to his partner—they can put the divisive anger and blame aside.

BEING AND DOING:
DIFFERENCES IN EMOTIONAL LANGUAGE

Therapists must be able to listen to clients on several levels. Especially in the field of family and marital therapy, clinicians have discovered how important it is to pay attention to nonverbal communication, to look at delivery (process) as well as content. In *Pragmatics of Human Communication*, now considered one of the classic works in family therapy literature, Watzlawick, Beavin, and Jackson (1967) demonstrate the value of studying the discrepancies in language as a means of understanding dysfunctional communication. Complex patterns of verbal and nonverbal language characterize most daily communications. Regardless of the level of complexity, the authors present several basic axioms about communication. Although these rules do not incorporate the influence of gender, the premise "one cannot not communicate" is particularly relevant to this discussion, and men are no exception. But there are additional rules that restrict what men are allowed to verbalize.

Men develop a language of logic and reason. Rationality and control become the cornerstones of their language. In the workplace this enables them to meet other's expectations and succeed. This is not something men learn from books, nor do they get instructions from family on appropriate verbal communication. During the long and complex process of gender-role socialization, men develop this manner of verbal expression without realizing the limitations it imposes on them. Intimate relationships with women is where these shortcomings are most painfully felt. Men learn not only how to express themselves, but when to. If we agree that men cannot readily communicate on intimate terms, then how do men learn to express their emotions? There is a metalanguage that develops from the restrictions of masculinity. It is gender-biased and gender-influenced, learned and practiced more by males than females. It is a language that is poorly understood by both men and women.

Given what men learn from the powerful social and cultural messages about manhood, we must now ask about how men communicate their emotional needs and wants. As indicated earlier, men become adept at denying their emotional needs. They find ways of getting these needs met without having to acknowledge they have them. Typically, a man's language does not contain statements such as, "I need to be close," or "I'm lonely," or "I'm feeling overwhelmed; I need time with you." As stated earlier, sexual intimacy is one means men can satisfy these needs. Some men can also express themselves through cooperative actions, if not words. A couple I saw recently provides an excellent example of this.

Ira and Liz, a childless couple in their mid-30s, went on a long-awaited weekend vacation to Vermont to escape from the pressures of work. Excited but exhausted from the week, they discussed how to spend the rest of the day. Liz stretched out on the large king-size bed, suggesting they just sit and talk for awhile. Ira immediately reached for the scrabble game and invited Liz to play. She showed little enthusiasm, but Ira, an avid game player, tried to talk her into it. Liz turned to Ira and, in a tone of voice displaying considerable displeasure, told Ira how upset she was by his suggestion. She let him know that just when they have some time to talk and be close, he wants to do something that will get in the way. The gist of Liz's comments, as we later reconstructed them, was that Ira's suggestion felt to her like he was distancing himself at a time when she wanted to get closer. The more they talked, the more heated things got, until finally Ira left in disgust. He felt angry and hurt, but was not sure why. Confused and frustrated, he took a walk to collect this thoughts.

Once alone, Ira realized that for him playing a game with Liz was a way to feel close to her. Yet Liz had always interpreted this as a desire to be distant, completely the opposite of what he intended. Excited by this important revelation, he returned to talk to Liz about it. This interesting discovery explained a number of the many breakdowns in their communication. When Liz could just be with Ira, she felt close. Ira felt close to Liz when he had any opportunity to do something with her. Being and doing is a distinction that highlights the difference in language learned by Ira and Liz through their gender-role conditioning.

"Being" and "doing" are concepts originally introduced by Chodorow (1971, 1978), who convincingly argues that gender socialization is largely responsible for the different languages men and women speak. Chodorow believes boys are more thoroughly taught to be masculine than girls are to be feminine; thus, the pressure on men is greater. With boys, intimate connections are likely to involve athletic activities and game playing. But whatever the activity, Chodorow (1978) believes that "masculine identification processes stress differentiation from others, denial of affective relation" and processes that "tend to deny the relationship" (p. 176).

Do men deny relationships, or is it that they make connections outside of the affective sphere? Liz regarded her husband's attempt to be intimate as spurious, leaving Ira feeling inadequate. Yet social and family influences have supported men's laconic style of communication, and, consequently, men do not feel there is anything wrong with this. It only becomes problematic when a man's partner asks him to acknowledge well-insulated parts of himself.

A man's emotional language becomes something other than a language of words; actions reveal more of a man's needs. Ira and Liz employ two very different "emotional languages." In Vermont, they both desired the same thing—closeness—yet their means of communicating this resulted in the opposite. When men are unable to express their needs in the same way as their partner, they can feel not only misunderstood but disbelieved. Men in positions similiar to Ira feel hurt, angry, and, even, unloved.

Of course, anger is the one strong emotion men typically express. Anger is the one emotion most men have observed in other men, particularly their fathers, which naturally results from the ongoing self-denial so common among men. But behind the mask of anger are other emotions that men deny. This emotional restrictiveness can lead to frustrating and unproductive marital struggles. Exchanges of anger are typically followed by mutual blaming, which leads each partner into defensive and self-protective postures. The utter frustration that many feel is demonstrated in the following clinical vignette. This couple decided that therapy might help them cope with the frustrations of infertility, which, after 3 years, was now generating more tension than they could handle alone:

WIFE: This discussion is beginning to get to me, I can't talk with him about this anymore. I mean, there's no support (pause), and I feel so alone . . . (starts to cry) . . . it's our problem, but it feels like only my problem.

THERAPIST: What happens to you when you try to discuss it with him?

WIFE: Well, it's extremely frustrating to try and discuss my feelings with someone who doesn't react . . . besides, he has to feel something—I can't believe he doesn't—but nothing ever shows.

HUSBAND: Wait a second, Susan, I've told you I feel sad about this—I feel real sad (This is said without any change in voice tone or facial expression). You know how much I've been looking forward to having a kid. But we can't dwell on this so much. (Turns to the therapist) You see, I know it will happen, and I try to reassure Susan so she'll settle down. She gets too emotional; it's not helping the situation at all.

WIFE: (Looking more upset) Just listen to this; this is exactly what I've been talking about. (She begins to cry again) I'm sorry, but this is so frustrating for me. I feel like such an idiot, crying here and feeling so badly, and he sits there and says I'm dwelling too much on how I feel. Dammit, I have a right to dwell on it, this is what I feel, and I need him to be there to talk about it with me. He sits there and acts so cool, so calm. I wonder if he really feels anything, I wonder how much he really wants this baby.

THERAPIST: What makes you question whether Art feels what he says he feels? He just said a moment ago that this was very sad for him as well.

WIFE: Look at him; he doesn't look sad at all. He talks so logically about it, it's sickening (sounding very angry). He hasn't shed a tear since we've been coming here . . . that's why I think he says he's sad—just because I feel this way; maybe he says it to appease me.

HUSBAND: (Looking visibly irritated) I'm getting really annoyed now. (Turns to the therapist) It really pisses me off when she does this. It seems like I have to cry in order for her to believe I feel sad . . . I'm not the kind of person who is outwardly emotional like her, so . . .

WIFE: Well, at least I'd know you're feeling something.

HUSBAND: But I do feel something; I feel lots of things. I get sick and tired of you telling me that I have to show feelings like you do; you know I don't express my emotions in that way. I never have and probably never will.

WIFE: I'm not interested in changing you, Art, but I would like some support. I'd like to talk with you without feeling that I'm some emotional freak, but you don't listen to me—that's one of our biggest problems. Whenever I try to talk with you, either you get into that real logical crap or you leave. How are we supposed to have a relationship when you do that?

HUSBAND: I feel sometimes that the only way you'll be satisfied with our relationship is if I become like you. I don't understand this, why can't I say I feel something in my own way. I listen to you; I just don't say things to you in the way you do. Sometimes I wonder if I can ever please you.

WIFE: What would please me, Art, would be having more time to talk with each other, like we are now.

THERAPIST: You know, I'm beginning to get a pretty good idea as to why you two don't get the time to talk. If this is any indication of what happens, I can appreciate why you don't get together. You both get real frustrated and angry, and neither of you feels very understood by the other, but I think one of the problems is that each of you has your own way of expressing what you feel—maybe because you feel things differently. You know, it's as if you're speaking different languages to each other.

WIFE: I can't believe you're saying that, because that's exactly what I said to my girlfriend the other day. She has the same problem with communication with her husband.

The source of Art's anger is not only Susan, although he does feel angry at not being understood. Art is angry because his language is different from Susan's, and he has not learned or been allowed as a man to speak her language. Here the therapist must help the couple recognize that their problem is neither her fault nor his. As we will discuss in the treatment section of this book, the therapist's task, among many, is to provide the couple with a new level of understanding so they can begin to listen to the other without blame and point out that neither's expressive style is the "right way" or "better way."

BUILDING BRIDGES

Art and Susan, like other couples whose plights are described in this chapter, have considerable difficulty understanding each other's needs. They cannot discuss their differences without producing more tension and emotional distance between them. While all but one of the couples mentioned here were seen in marital therapy, their patterns of interaction are prevalent among many heterosexual couples.

This chapter has attempted to show that men are conditioned to act in ways that work against healthy marital interaction. In addition, fundamental differences exist in their expression of affection, what they reveal, and how they present themselves socially. Most importantly, we have tried to demonstrate that both genders lack a critical understanding of how the other has been conditioned to think, feel, and behave according to gender-biased rules, and how this impacts on their relationship.

The intensity of this gender-based conflict has been heightened by the Women's Movement and the Men's Movement. Women such as Lorraine, whom we discussed in the beginning of the chapter, 20 years ago might have felt not only tentative and guilty about striking out to establish a career and life outside the family, they would have also felt socially alienated and unsupported by female peers. Not only were resources for women scarce, there was also a prevailing social attitude that women were abandoning their families if they worked outside the home. Women today are, in general, more confident and flexible in letting go of the hold that traditional roles have had on them. Ironically, today a woman is more likely to feel unsupported in the traditional role of full-time caretaker due to the declining numbers of women remaining at home. The Women's Movement has clearly been a source of support for women who wish to expand their lives.

The Men's Movement, on the other hand, is still in its infancy, unsure of its footing and without a clear, consistent sense of direction. Men such as Lorraine's husband Harry are trying desperately to understand what they are supposed to do. Many are trying to be more flexible, sensitive, and supportive. But for the most part, these men operate without adequate role models or support from male peers. Most men live in a social environment today that parallels that of the early Women's Movement in that men who attempt to escape from the traditional mold receive mixed messages, at best. From their male peers, husbands receive little support and guidance, and at times even derision when they attempt to change work and leisure priorities in order to accommodate their wives.

The men who want to alter relationships that are based on traditional roles are still a minority. These men generally struggle alone, trying to adapt to the changes of their female mates—alone because such men do not commonly confide in anyone other than their mates, and alone because most men do not feel part of any movement they can embrace.

Perhaps the most obvious effect of the different stages of the Men's and Women's Movements is that women are generally supported in their open display of dissatisfaction with men and tend to be more assertive and confident when doing so. Most men do not feel part of a movement and lack a context of support for their reactions to frustrated mates. In therapy we frequently hear men complain that they feel "damned if they do and damned if they don't" in their attempts to become more open and expressive. One man aptly put it this way, "When I try to be more open and sensitive, I'm criticized for not doing it well enough, and when I stop trying in order to avoid criticism, I'm condemned for that."

It is important for both sexes to recognize where the other is in their development, and try to respond accordingly. It is critical that each gender understand how its own changes and lack of changes affects the other. Just as women have had to struggle with the discomfort of carving out new roles that contrast with the ones their mothers taught them, men must also contend with the discomfort of altering the roles they were taught.

In most instances, adult men today see their fathers' experience as a pattern of home life which defined the way relationships should be conducted. The male partner often feels that he is losing something: giving up what his father had and what his father's father would likely describe as a perfectly logical arrangement between a husband and wife. Concomitant with the sense of, "Dad didn't have to do this kind of stuff; why do I?," is the challenge to one's "masculinity." How comfortable will a man be with himself if he does something his father would regard as unmanly?

Our clinical experience tells us not to underestimate the power these internalized messages have on a man's expectations of himself as a husband. While men are trying to accommodate to the changes in women, they inevitably find it a tremendous challenge to their masculine identity.

The traditional male role afforded men a position in their families that was comfortable, not only because it was familiar, but also because it offered clear ways to experience self-worth and validation. Men were rewarded for what they felt they did best—being the family breadwinner and provider of security. Compared to their wives, men saw themselves doing the harder job, waging daily "battles" to be sure the family had enough to eat, a nice home, and suitable clothing. In turn, they were typically rewarded for their efforts by being nurtured by their wives and remained free of domestic obligations.

With more women now entering the work force, men find themselves in a quandary. It is no longer enough for a husband to perform as the breadwinner and rest on his laurels at home. Men no longer receive accolades for only fulfilling that role, which has been central to their identity. As wives work outside of the home and become less available to fill their husbands' needs, husbands feel abandoned: Their wives are not there to nurture and provide for them as in the past. As a result of these major changes, husbands feel unsettled, confused, and sometimes shocked by the demands of changing roles and expectations.

The men cited in the examples represent the kind of frustration common among many married men. In general, they feel misunderstood and betrayed, as though somehow they can never do enough. Scarf (1987) cites an example of a husband who worked three jobs for a long period of time without realizing the toll on him, his family, and his marriage. Because men see this as their duty, they may not be aware of the negative consequences of being so driven. Scarf (1987) quotes this man as saying "'I didn't think of myself as mean, . . . I perceived myself entirely differently—as a good person, very harassed, yet doing his best for his family's welfare'" (p. 345).

Most men have not relinquished the notion that being a provider and competing at work to provide security for their families is their most important function. Even when his wife contributes a significant portion of the family income, a husband may not relieve himself of the pressures to provide. He views his income as still the critical one—a view often based in reality but almost always in emotions as well. Thus, men still bear the strain of feeling they are ultimately responsible for the family's welfare. Because women are similarly conditioned to see men as providers, they can unwittingly reinforce this male attitude about being economically responsible.

With this provider role still central to their male self-image, in addition to a whole new array of expectations for support and involvement, many men now feel as stressed at home as they do at work. They believe they cannot do enough to win over their wives. They are still seeking the kind of admiration from a woman that reinforces their masculinity and lets them feel like a hero. Unable to secure this feminine recognition, many of the husbands we have talked with throw up their hands and wonder if they will ever please their wives and be successful as husbands. As a result, men often withdraw and turn to someone or something that will insulate them from their hurt and disappointment. Men unable to contain their aggressive impulses inflict on their partners the kind of repetitious confrontations and violence that occur with alarming frequency.

To move beyond the emotional and structural stalemate men and women find themselves in today requires a whole new level of understanding. When Susan and Art discover they are speaking different languages, that becomes the basis for change. It is easy to assume we are understood by others, especially those who are close to us. Their responses are frequently taken as confirmation of what we want to believe. In fact, most men and women do not feel completely understood by their partner. A critical step in transcending this problem is recognizing that men and women have different modes of expressing their feelings. Furthermore, there can be great disparity in their ability to empathize with the other because of the different roles they learned about relationships.

Learning the differences in how we relate to feelings, without judging the other as wrong, malicious, or inept can help to deal with these differences constructively and without blame. The dominant message to men from the Women's Movement has been one of criticism and judgment, with little consideration for sources of the problem. Kolbenschlag (1979), in her letter to the Frog Prince, and to men in general, says, "You haven't learned the art of living." This kind of judgment suggests that women's ways of living are all wise and on target, while men are totally adrift from living life the right way. Such a statement not only distorts, but drives a wedge between men and women every bit as much as the message that men send to women about being weak and incompetent. If women buy into the notion that they have learned the art of living and men have not, they will be less likely to listen to men and try to understand them and their differences.

If men and women believe that they must learn each other's languages, and that neither has the sole possession of The True Way Of Life, then it becomes possible to begin building bridges to each other. There is much that is necessary to overcome the tension and misunderstanding between the genders. A therapeutic framework for change, with a more detailed analysis of how to surmount the obstacles to change for men, is presented in the concluding chapters of this book. We present here three critical elements essential to any change process between the genders as a concluding summary:

1. *Expectations*: Both genders must examine the attitudes and expectations they have of each other with respect to their roles, their needs, and the needs of the other. Each gender must also examine how they unconsciously contribute to locking the other into the very patterns they dislike.

2. *Seeing the Real Conflicts*: The genders cannot achieve meaningful understanding without looking beneath the surface to what is at stake emotionally. Instead of seeing men as unwilling to change or women as impossible to satisfy, we must look for such emotional reactions as fear of change; response to giving up familiar and comforting habits; and fear of rejection, failure, and dependency, even though these may be unacknowledged.

3. *Differentiation*: Each gender must recognize and be responsible for its own emotional baggage, its own needs and choices, and how they have sought to deal with these. Women cannot be responsible for creating the changes men need to make, but they will also block those changes from happening if they cannot accept men's right to change in their own ways.

All of these changes will take time. They involve painful discarding and relearning. We must let go of many of the powerful messages about masculinity and femininity. By reeducating ourselves and each other we can begin to replace blame with mutual understanding and respect, so men and women can coexist in more peaceful and satisfying ways.

REFERENCES

Bell, D. (1982). *Being a man: the paradox of masculinity*. San Diego: Harcourt Brace Jovanovich.

Chodorow, N. (1971). Being and doing: a cross-cultural examination of the socialization of males and females. In V. Gornick and B. Moran (Eds.), *Woman in sexist society: Studies in power and powerlessness*. New York: Basic Books.

Chodorow, N. (1978). *The reproduction of mothering.* Berkeley, CA: University of California Press.

Farrell, W. (1986). *Why men are the way they are.* New York: McGraw-Hill.

Gilligan, C. (1982). *In a different voice.* Cambridge, MA: Harvard University Press.

Kazantzakis, N. (1952). *Zorba the Greek.* New York: Simon & Schuster.

Kolbenschlag, M. (1979). *Kiss Sleeping Beauty good-bye: Breaking the spell of feminine myths and models.* Garden City, NY: Doubleday.

Monick, E. (1987). *Phallos: Sacred image of the masculine.* Toronto: Inner City Books.

Osherson, S. (1986). *Finding our fathers.* New York: Free Press.

Rubin, L. (1983). *Intimate strangers.* New York: Harper & Row.

Scarf, M. (1988). *Intimate partners.* New York: Ballantine Books.

Watzlawick, P., Beavin, J., & Jackson, D. (1967). *Pragmatics of human communication.* New York: W. W. Norton.

·4·

Fathers and Fathering

LARRY B. FELDMAN

Traditionally, the father role has been defined by two major characteristics: (1) being a good economic provider, and (2) being a firm disciplinarian. Nurturant child care has been defined as the mother's domain and, therefore, not an expected or valued activity for fathers (Feldman, 1982).

Based on this traditional role definition, fathers have generally been much less involved than mothers in the day-to-day care of their children (Kotelchuck, 1976; Pleck, 1979). When they have become involved, it has most often been in the role of disciplinarian. This role fits the masculine stereotype that men should be strong, tough, and aggressive in their dealings with other people, including their children. Consistent with this mode of structuring the father–child relationship, children have typically experienced their fathers as more punitive and less nurturing than their mothers (Feldman, 1982).

Low father involvement in nurturant parenting and rigidly traditional (authoritarian and punitive) fathering impede the development of children's self-esteem, frustration tolerance, impulse control, cognitive functioning, and interpersonal relationships (Biller, 1982). Children experience lack of father involvement as rejection; they experience paternal rigidity and punitiveness as condemnation. These reactions undermine the development of self-acceptance and self-esteem and stimulate feelings of frustration and helplessness. When the degree of "paternal deprivation" is severe, children and adolescents manifest a high incidence of behavior control problems, drug or alcohol abuse, and depression (Biller, 1982).

The traditional father role also impedes the psychological development of fathers. The experience of nurturing, supporting, and guiding children provides men with a unique opportunity to develop and fulfill their generative potential. Failure to actualize this potential creates a void in the emotional lives of a great many fathers. This void was described in the following way by a father who spent a rare morning taking care of his daughter while his wife was out of town: "I felt wonderful while I was taking care of her. Afterward, however, I felt very depressed when I thought about how seldom we are together and how little we know each other." Similar feelings are often expressed by divorced fathers who have little contact with their children. Such men have a very high incidence of psychiatric symptoms, particularly anxiety and depression. In fact, the best predictor of a divorced father's psychological adjustment is the amount of involvement that he has with his children (Jacobs, 1982).

BARRIERS TO NURTURANT FATHERING

What are the factors that inhibit men from actively participating in the nurturant care of their children? Answers to this question can be found at two levels: intrapsychic and interpersonal.

Intrapsychic Barriers

At the intrapsychic level, one major barrier to active parenting by men is anxiety (conscious and unconscious) stemming from traditional gender-role socialization (Feldman, 1982). From an early age, men are conditioned to fear being viewed as "feminine." They are also conditioned to view child care as a "feminine" activity. Therefore, active participation in child care is a potent stimulus for anxiety. An example of this anxiety is provided by Fein (1974), who describes the experience of a truck driver who was invited by his son's nursery school teacher to spend a morning with the class. After much hesitation, he agreed to come and ended up having a wonderful time playing with and reading a story to the children. As he was leaving, he turned to the teacher and thanked him for extending the invitation. However, he then got a puzzled, anxious look on his face and said, "What'll I tell the guys at work about this?" The anxiety expressed in this man's face and words is a reflection of the inhibitory power of the male gender-role injunction forbidding "feminine" behavior. This injunction is a major barrier to active, involved fathering.

A second source of anxiety about active fathering is fear of failure. Many men feel insecure about their ability to function competently as nurturers and are afraid they will be humiliated if they make the effort. This fear is reinforced by media images of men making bumbling and unsuccessful efforts to care for children, especially young children (a recent example is the movie *Three Men and a Baby*). Research studies have found that low father involvement in parenting is associated with low perceived skill at child-care tasks (McHale & Huston, 1984; Russell & Radin, 1983). The perception of incompetence leads to fear of failure and humiliation. These feelings, in turn, lead to avoidance of nurturant parenting.

The most deeply rooted intrapsychic barriers to father involvement in nurturant child care are derived from men's experiences in their families of origin. One such barrier stems from the importance of identification with the father as a mechanism by which boys develop a sense of self-cohesion and self-esteem. Since, at this time, most men's fathers were minimally involved in parenting, this is the model with which they have identified. Behaving in ways that are substantially different from the model, i.e., becoming a highly involved parent, threatens this identification and stimulates conscious or unconscious anxiety. For example, a 35-year-old psychologist is torn between his desire to be actively involved in parenting his 5-year-old son and his fear of being viewed by his business-oriented father as a "poor provider" if he takes large amounts of time away from his practice for parenting. He also fears that his father will be threatened if he sees his son being a "better father" than he was. As a result of these anxieties, he inhibits his desire to parent, works long hours in his practice, and feels depressed about the lack of a deeper relationship with his son.

In addition to the pressure to identify with an uninvolved father, men must also cope with the fact that because they were parented primarily by their mothers, their original identification was with a member of the opposite sex. A number of theorists (Chodorow, 1978; Dinnerstein, 1976; Rubin, 1983) have suggested that this arrangement stimulates a great deal of anxiety in young boys because it threatens their emerging sense of gender identity. Over time, this anxiety leads to the development of a defensive need to maintain rigid interpersonal boundaries. For many men, this need persists into adulthood. Since nurturant parenting, especially with infants and young children, requires boundary flexibility rather than rigidity, this situation becomes a potent stimulus for male anxiety. This anxiety is generally dealt with by avoidance of the potentially anxiety-provoking situation.

Interpersonal Barriers

At the interpersonal level, one factor that exerts an inhibitory effect on more involved parenting by fathers is the overt or covert expression of ambivalence by mothers. On one hand, many women want their husbands to be more involved in parenting so that they can be relieved of role overload and the children can have a better relationship with their father. On the other hand, there is often a good deal of anxiety, guilt, and resentment about giving up the role of "primary parent." These feelings may lead to excluding or critical behaviors that undermine the father's efforts to become more involved. For example, the father may be excluded from important decision-making processes (scheduling school conferences, planning after-school activities, etc.), he may be criticized when his parenting style differs from that of his wife, or his ability to effectively handle child-care responsibilities may be repeatedly questioned.

In divorced families, where the father is the noncustodial parent 90% of the time, hostility and conflict between the parents is often a major impediment to father involvement. Some fathers withdraw from their children in order to avoid conflict with their ex-wives. Other fathers are blocked in their efforts to be involved with their children by overt or covert interference from the mother (e.g., scheduling medical appointments or music lessons during the father's parenting time) (Hodges, 1986).

Outside of the family, work-related pressure represents a substantial barrier to involved fathering. Employers are generally highly resistant to the idea of men wanting to make adjustments in their work schedules or work hours in order to take care of their children. In one study (Rosen, Jerdee, & Prestwich, 1975), 1500 employers were asked to read a memorandum (created for the purpose of the study) from an employee requesting a 1-month unpaid leave of absence in order to care for his or her three young children. In the memos read by half of the employers, the employee requesting the leave was a woman; in those read by the other half, the employee was a man. The request for leave was perceived as significantly less appropriate when it came from a male employee than when it came from a female employee. Also, the employers were significantly less likely to grant such a leave to a man than to a woman.

The effect of such attitudes on the behavior of male employees is illustrated by the experience of Swedish workers. In Sweden there is a national policy requiring employers to offer 6 months of paid parental leave, divided between the parents at their discretion. In spite of this policy, very few Swedish men (approximately 10%) take any parental leave, and those who do take very little (less than 2 months). When questioned about their reasons for not taking parental leave, Swedish men most often stated that they were afraid their employers would disapprove and that sanctions would be imposed if they took this option (Lamb & Levine, 1983).

EFFECTS OF INCREASED FATHER INVOLVEMENT

Despite the internal and external barriers to nurturant fathering, some fathers do become highly involved in child care. Recently, a number of research studies have begun to examine the correlates of more involved fathering for children, fathers, and mothers.

Children

Three studies of intact families have directly assessed children with highly involved fathers and compared their development with that of children whose fathers are less involved in parenting. In a study of infants (2–22 months old) with fathers giving primary care, Pruett (1987) found no negative effects and a number of positive ones. In general, the infants were developing well in all areas and showed above-average development of cognitive and social skills. Radin (1982) studied a group of 3- to 6-year-old children in the United States and compared those with fathers giving equal or primary care with those whose fathers were less involved in child care. Radin found a positive association between high father involvement and the development of (1) internal locus of control, a measure of the degree to which children feel in control of their lives, and (2) cognitive ability, particularly in the verbal area. In addition, there was a negative correlation between high father involvement and stereotyped perceptions of parental roles; i.e., the more involved the fathers, the less stereotyped were the children's perceptions. Sagi (1982) utilized

Radin's basic research design with a sample of Israeli families of 3- to 6-year-old children. As in the study in the United States, children whose fathers were highly involved in fathering had a more developed sense of internal locus of control and a less stereotyped view of parental roles. In addition, these children also showed a higher degree of empathy than did children with less involved fathers.

The results of these studies clearly suggest that high father involvement in nurturant parenting is beneficial for children's development. The benefits include both traditionally "masculine" attributes (e.g., internal locus of control) and traditionally "feminine" attributes (e.g., empathy). In addition, this arrangement appears to inhibit the development of gender-role stereotyping. In all of the studies, high father involvement was equally beneficial for girls and boys.

In divorced families, high father involvement has been studied in families with joint-custody and father-custody arrangements. Studies of children in joint-custody families (e.g., Abarbanel, 1979; Luepnitz, 1982; Steinman, 1981) have indicated that most children adjust well and appear to benefit from the high level of father involvement. A distinct advantage of the joint custody arrangement is that children do not experience the loss of a meaningful relationship with their fathers, an outcome that is not uncommon in mother-custody families (Hetherington & Hagan, 1986).

Studies of father-custody families have generally reported no significant differences overall between children living in father-custody and mother-custody homes (Santrock & Warshak, 1986). However, some studies (e.g., Santrock, Warshak, & Elliot, 1982) have found significant relationships among the sex of the child, the sex of the custodial parent, and the child's social, emotional, and cognitive development. All other things being equal, boys tend to do better in father-custody homes and girls tend to do better in mother-custody homes.

Fathers and Father–Child Relationships

Most fathers who become highly involved in the care of their children report an increase in their understanding of and sensitivity to their children's needs, an increase in the closeness of their relationships with their children, and an increase in their enjoyment of the time they spend with their children. They also report feeling more self-confident and more effective as parents (Russell, 1986).

On the other hand, highly involved fathers also report an increase in the level of conflict between them and their children, probably as a result of the increased contact and increased responsibility for day-to-day activities. Despite this increased level of conflict, most of these fathers describe increased feelings of satisfaction with their parental role (Russell & Radin, 1983).

Mothers and Mother–Child Relationships

For mothers as well as fathers, the effects of increased father involvement in parenting are mostly positive. Role overload is reduced, feelings of autonomy and self-esteem increase, and anxiety about leaving child care in the hands of strangers is eliminated (Hoffman, 1983; Russell, 1986). However, a substantial minority of mothers in shared-caregiving families also report a good deal of dissatisfaction with their reduced contact and influence on their children and a good deal of concern about the quality of their husband's parenting (Russell, 1986).

DEVELOPMENTAL ASPECTS OF FATHERING

In both traditional (low father involvement) and nontraditional (high father involvement) families, the nature of the fathering experience changes during the various stages of a child's development. Each stage presents new challenges, new responsibilities, and new opportunities for positive growth in the father–child relationship.

Infancy

In the traditional family, the father's primary role during infancy is to be an economic and emotional support to the mother so that she can comfortably form a close, "symbiotic" bond with the baby (Mahler, Pine, & Bergman, 1975). As the infant matures the father takes on an additional role, that of the "second other," who helps the child begin to separate and individuate from the mother by providing an alternative source of stimulation for his or her burgeoning exploratory drive. However, when the infant becomes fearful and seeks a temporary regression to symbiotic dependency, the mother again becomes the primary attachment figure (Mahler, Pine, & Bergman, 1975).

In the nontraditional family, where the father is highly involved in parenting, a different set of relationship dynamics develop. Here, there is a "dual symbiosis" (Abelin, 1975), with a high degree of attachment between the infant and the father as well as the mother. In this type of family, when the infant enters the stage of separation-individuation, each parent provides a secure base from which the infant can explore his or her world and to which the infant can return when (s)he needs a temporary regression.

Preschool Period (3–5 Years of Age)

During the preschool years, gender identity is established, and boys and girls begin to develop somewhat different relationships with their fathers. This is the period of the "family romance," when children typically form a romantic attachment with the opposite-sex parent and a rivalrous relationship with the same-sex parent. Thus, girls begin to exhibit flirtatious and possessive behavior toward their fathers while boys become competitive and excluding.

Ideally, fathers are able to deal with these developments without becoming overly anxious, angry, or sexually stimulated. In some instances, however, fathers' reactions are dysfunctional. With girls, some fathers become so anxious about the flirtatiousness that they withdraw or are rejecting. Other fathers, whose personalities are characterized by low self-esteem, low frustration tolerance, and poor impulse control, may become sexually abusive during this period of time (Thorman, 1983). With boys, some fathers react to the competitive behavior with anger and hostility. Others become discouraged and withdrawn. All of these dysfunctional reactions impair the child's ability to develop a healthy sense of self-esteem by depriving him or her of the opportunity to experience a warm, loving, accepting, and admiring father who is able to maintain appropriate intergenerational boundaries without needing to either withdraw or attack.

In families with more highly involved fathers, the sex differences associated with this period of development are less pronounced than in the traditional family. Because of the father's more active involvement in parenting, girls are less likely to experience him as a distant, romantic ideal, and boys are less likely to experience him as a competitive rival. Based on the existing data (e.g., Pruett, 1987; Russell & Radin, 1983), the attenuation of these sex differences does not appear to be harmful to children's development and may, in fact, be helpful. At the very least, it diminishes the development of gender-role stereotyping.

Juvenile Period (6–12 Years of Age)

When children enter school their attention becomes highly focused on formal learning for much of the day. One factor that is clearly associated with successful academic achievement is active father involvement in parenting. In traditional families this association is stronger for boys than for girls (Radin, 1981), perhaps because fathers in traditional families often view academic achievement as less important for girls than for boys. Studies of nontraditional, shared-parenting families of school-aged children are not yet available; however, the existing studies of families with young children have not found a sex difference in the association between father involvement and cognitive development. Girls and boys both appear to benefit from the increase in father's cognitive stimulation (Russell & Radin, 1983). One probable explanation for this lack of sex difference is that fathers who become highly involved in child care are likely to view academic achievement as being equally as important for girls as it is for boys.

Adolescence (13–19 Years of Age)

During the adolescent years, fathers are faced with a host of new issues and conflicts as they attempt to cope with their son's or daughter's burgeoning autonomy and sexuality. As the adolescent matures, the father's affection, support, and guidance are important resources promoting healthy development. Fathers need to be empathically attuned to the adolescent's shifting needs for dependency and autonomy and be able to adjust their behavior as these needs change over time. This is often difficult for fathers to do because male role conditioning is so heavily oriented toward the importance of domination and control. As a result, conflict between fathers and teenage children is common, especially with boys. Most fathers are able to develop sufficient understanding and flexibility to work through these conflicts and help their son or daughter grow into adulthood. Some, however, become hostile or abusive, while others withdraw and have little or no interaction with their adolescent. In these situations, the likelihood of the teenager developing one or more of a variety of social, emotional, and academic problems is high (Martin, 1985).

CLINICAL IMPLICATIONS

Types of Dysfunctional Father–Child Relationships

Insufficient and/or dysfunctional fathering are major factors leading to the development of behavioral or emotional problems in children, fathers, and families. In this section, the most frequent types of dysfunctional father–child relationships will be described and illustrated with clinical examples.

Disengagement

The most common dysfunctional pattern is disengagement, with the father having little or no involvement in the child's day-to-day life. Lack of father involvement is experienced by children as rejection and impairs the development of self-esteem. Clinically, this is most often manifested in the form of depression and/or conduct disorder.

Example. The divorced mother of a 13-year-old boy ("Andy") requested therapy because of her son's oppositional behavior at school (his grades were extremely poor because he would not do homework or study for tests) and at home (he refused to participate in household chores and was extremely irritable and argumentative). Father was peripheral; he visited once or twice a month (irregularly) and phoned occasionally.

During the initial evaluation interviews, it quickly became apparent that Andy harbored a great deal of resentment toward his father for being "the cause of the divorce" and for "abandoning" him after the divorce. His passive-aggressive behavior was, to a large degree, a way of getting his father's attention and expressing his resentment toward him. Intrapsychically, he was struggling with painful feelings of worthlessness and helplessness, deriving to a large degree from his perception that his father did not love or value him.

Father expressed concern about his son's behavioral problems and criticized his wife for not "disciplining" him more effectively. He perceived himself as too busy with his work to be able to spend as much time with his son as he would like to.

In the therapy, Andy was able to talk with his father about some of his feelings of resentment and anger. Father was initially defensive but over time was able to empathize with his son's underlying pain and longing for a relationship with him. He began to increase the frequency of his phone calls and visits. Initially, Andy was resistant to these initiatives, experiencing them as "too little, too late." Eventually, he softened, and the father–son relationship began to improve. As this happened, Andy's oppositional behavior diminished, and his mood improved.

Conflict

A second type of dysfunctional father–child relationship is characterized by the father playing the role of the "heavy" whose interactions with his child are primarily related to being a disciplinarian. This pattern is usually associated with behavior control problems, often of an aggressive nature.

Example. Ten-year-old "Bill" and his parents were referred for family therapy because of Bill's aggressive behavior (verbal and physical) in school and at home. The father's role in this family was primarily that of disciplinarian. When mother became frustrated with Bill's behavior, she called her husband at work and asked him to come home and "do something" with their son. Father would then come home and attempt to discipline his son. Often, this led to verbal, and sometimes physical, battles between Bill and his father.

It soon became apparent that these "disciplinary actions" by father were the predominant form of interaction between him and his son. There were very few positive experiences. In the therapy, this began to change. Father was encouraged to invite Bill to do things with him that he thought they both might enjoy. At first, these were very tense experiences; neither Bill nor father felt comfortable just "being together." Conversation was difficult and strained; often, there were long periods of silence. Over time, however, they began to relax and were able to share some positive moments together. These experiences seemed to have a soothing effect on Bill. His behavior became less aggressive at school and at home, and he reported feeling less anxious and more content. Father's mood also improved. He felt frustrated and angry much less often and felt increasingly positive about his changing relationship with his son.

Coalition

A third pattern of dysfunctional father–child interaction is characterized by an overt or covert cross-generational coalition between father and child. This pattern is more common with daughters than with sons.

Example. A 15-year-old girl ("Carol") and her family came for therapy because of Carol's depressed mood and the extremely frequent conflict between Carol and her mother. Father's role was that of peacemaker between his wife and daughter. Carol complained to her father when she felt her mother was being unreasonable. Father then spoke to mother to try to get things straightened out. Mother felt undermined in her efforts to discipline her daughter. Father felt frustrated and confused. Carol felt depressed.

In therapy, the parents were helped to restructure their relationship with their daughter. Mother asked father to take more responsibility for dealing with Carol's behavioral problems (not doing homework, coming home after curfew, experimenting with alcohol and drugs). Father agreed to do this but asked mother, in turn, to reduce the frequency and intensity of her negative behavior with Carol (yelling, name-calling, threatening).

These changes were difficult to make at first because of underlying emotional issues in both parents. Father unconsciously enjoyed being a "hero" to his daughter and was reluctant to give up this role. Mother was unconsciously rivalrous with Carol and was acting out competitive, aggressive impulses in relation to her.

Over time, these dynamics began to shift. Father did assume more responsibility for discipline and began insisting that Carol discuss her feelings about her mother with her directly. Mother reduced the frequency and intensity of her hostile behavior toward Carol. These changes led to a reduction in conflict between Carol and her mother, and an improvement in Carol's behavior and mood. Tension between father and mother was reduced, and the relationship between father and Carol was transformed from a covert coalition to a positive relationship with appropriate intergenerational boundaries.

Abuse

The most extreme type of dysfunctional father–child relationship is one marked by physical or sexual abuse (or, in some instances, both).

Fathers are the identified offenders in approximately half of the reported cases of physical abuse and in the vast majority (over 90%) of reported sexual abuse cases (Jason, Burton, Williams, & Rochat, 1982).

Abusive fathers have generally been described as rigidly traditional, authoritarian men with low self-esteem, low frustration tolerance, and poor impulse control (Tyler, 1986). They also have little ability to empathize with the age-appropriate needs and capabilities of their children. An illustration of these dynamics in relation to physical abuse is provided by the comments of a father who had fractured the skull of his 18-month-old baby during punishment for a mistake in toilet training, "He knows better; he did it deliberately. I'll show him who's boss; who does he think he is anyway. . . . You have to teach kids to respect authority, otherwise they'll grow up spoiled rotten" (Steele, 1980, p. 486).

Sexually abusive fathers usually manifest a very high degree of denial, even when confronted with overwhelming evidence that they have been abusive (Mayer, 1983). When they do admit to the abuse, they often attempt to justify their behavior via rationalization. For example, one abusive father stated that his sexual involvement with his daughter was primarily a means of showing affection and that "I just wanted to be a good dad to her and have her like me" (Thorman, 1983, p. 38).

Herman (1981) has postulated that the marked discrepancy between the frequency of sexual abuse by fathers as compared to mothers is explainable to a large degree by the fact that men generally have had little or no involvement in the nurturant care of their young children. This hypothesis has received support from research indicating that men who are sexually abusive with their children have typically been less involved in the care of their children than men who have not been sexually abusive (Parker & Parker, 1986).

Fathers and Family Therapy

Just as fathers have generally been less involved than mothers in the process of parenting, they have also been less involved in the process of family therapy. Fathers seldom call to make an initial appointment for family therapy, often do not come for scheduled family therapy appointments, and usually demonstrate the most resistance to the continuation of the therapy once it has begun (Berg & Rosenblum,

1977; Shapiro & Budman, 1973). On the other hand, when fathers do actively participate and are willing to accept some of the responsibility for the family's problems, the likelihood of a positive outcome is high (Heubeck, Watson, & Russell, 1986).

Barriers to Father Involvement in Family Therapy

Intrapsychic Barriers. Male gender-role conditioning dictates that men should be strong and self-sufficient—when there are problems, a "real man" solves them himself. Asking others for help is a distinctly "nonmasculine" behavior. As a result, men are reluctant to seek psychotherapeutic help when they or their families are having problems.

In addition, fathers generally do not view themselves as having responsibility for their children's behavior problems (Watson, 1985). This denial of responsibility contrasts with the fact that change in the father–child relationship is a major predictor of positive outcome in family therapy (Heubeck, Watson, & Russell, 1986).

Interpersonal Barriers. The most important interpersonal barrier to fathers' involvement in family therapy is the therapist's or clinic's failure to include the father from the outset of the family therapy process. Often, when mothers call to make an initial appointment, no mention is made of the importance of father's participation. When this is mentioned, there is often an overt or covert message indicating that his presence is optional (e.g., "if possible, I would also like your husband to come"). Seldom are both parents included in the planning and scheduling of the initial appointment.

When parents are divorced, it is even easier for the father to be neglected, since he is almost always the noncustodial parent. However, the relationship between a symptomatic child and his or her noncustodial father is often of crucial importance in the assessment and treatment of the child's problems. When the therapist is clear about the importance of the noncustodial father and actively reaches out to include him from the beginning of the family therapy process, an important barrier to the father's participation is removed.

Another therapist-generated barrier to fathers' participation in family therapy is the therapist's manner of relating to the father during family therapy interviews. Often, fathers are the most resistant members of the family. If the therapist responds to the resistance with overt or covert hostility, the likelihood of the father returning for further interviews is diminished. On the other hand, if the therapist is able to accept the resistance as a defense against anxiety and finds a way to validate the father's importance to the family and the family therapy, the likelihood of his continuing participation is high.

Fathers and Individual Therapy

When divorced fathers come for individual psychotherapy, issues related to fathering are often in the foreground. In fact, the most difficult problem for most divorced fathers (90% of whom are noncustodial parents) is coping with feelings of anxiety and depression related to a sense of loss of their children (Jacobs, 1982). The most important therapeutic task with such men is to help them maintain as much contact as possible with their children and to develop positive postdivorce relationships with them (Jacobs, 1983).

When married fathers come for individual psychotherapy, problems related to the father–child relationship are seldom presented as a primary reason for seeking help. Nonetheless, it is important for therapists to keep in mind the possibility that issues related to parenting may be an important underlying dynamic theme. For example, a 30-year-old man came for individual therapy because of depression. One stimulus for his depression was financial pressure. He experienced himself as a failure (not a "good provider") because his income was not sufficient to meet his family's financial needs. The only solution that he could envision was to take a second job, even though that would mean spending very little time with his two young children, whom he cherished and enjoyed taking care of when he was not working. When the therapist inquired about the possibility of him asking his wife to share the provider role, he was highly ambivalent. He very much wanted to continue to be involved with his children but he felt guilty and ashamed about asking his wife to share something that he perceived as his responsibility. Ultimately, he did discuss this issue with his wife, and they worked out a role-sharing arrangement in which they both worked and both spent time caring for the children. Soon thereafter, his depression began to lift.

With all men in therapy, it is important to explore the emotional significance of their relationship with their own father. A great deal of the psychological distress that brings men to therapy is closely connected to feelings of deprivation or abuse in relation to their fathers. For example, a 41-year-old man came for psychotherapy because of anxiety and depression associated with the mid-life transition. During the course of his therapy he became acutely and painfully aware of how little attention, acceptance, or admiration he had received from his father and what a highly significant role that was playing in his current feelings of being a worthless failure, in spite of considerable objective success. No matter how much other people might admire or praise him, nothing could make up for the lack of affirmation that he had experienced in his relationship with his father. This theme became the major focus of his therapy.

REMOVING THE BARRIERS TO NURTURANT FATHERING

The task of removing the internal and external barriers to involved, nurturant fathering requires change at a variety of different levels. Intrapsychically, men need to overcome feelings of anxiety, shame, and guilt associated with stereotyped images of "masculine" and "feminine" behavior. They also need to overcome feelings of inadequacy based on the incorrect belief that men are not well-equipped to provide nurturant care because they do not have a "maternal instinct." Numerous studies have demonstrated that men are equally as capable as women of providing responsive, nurturant care for their children, including infants and very young children (Lamb, 1982; Parke, 1981). Other studies (e.g., Parke, Hymel, Power, & Tinsley, 1980) have indicated that training in child-care skills significantly increases the degree of men's involvement in nurturant parenting. Such training reduces fear of failure and humiliation, increases self-confidence, and stimulates a positive desire to participate in child-care activities.

At the interpersonal level, it is important that mothers support fathers' increased involvement in active parenting. This requires confronting and resolving feelings of ambivalence related to the importance of being the "primary parent" and identifying and changing behaviors that undermine fathers' efforts to become more involved in parenting.

When families come for therapy, it is essential that the therapist be aware of the importance of active, involved fathering for the well-being of children, fathers, and mothers. Fathers need to be included in the therapy process from the beginning and related to in such a way that their resistances are reduced rather than strengthened. Mothers need to be helped to reduce ambivalence about father involvement and to eliminate behaviors that undermine such involvement. Couples need to be helped to constructively negotiate mutually satisfactory agreements about parenting responsibilities and parenting styles.

In individual therapy with men who are fathers, feelings about fathering need to become a routine focus of assessment and, when indicated, therapeutic intervention. With all men, regardless of whether or not they are fathers, the crucial psychodynamic significance of their relationship with their own father should always be a major dimension of therapeutic exploration.

Therapists can also contribute to the removal of barriers to nurturant fathering by stimulating changes in society. In the workplace, it is essential that men be given the opportunity to take parental leave when a baby is born, to have access to a flexible work schedule so that family needs can be coordinated with work needs, and to be able to work a limited number of hours per week so that sufficient time is available for parenting (see Pleck, 1986, for more on this issue). Equally, if not more, important is the necessity for change in the attitudes of employers and employees toward the idea of a man wanting to be highly involved in parenting his children. It is essential that men stop being placed in a position where the only way to succeed in their job is to neglect their family.

In the educational arena, children must be given the message that child care is a desirable and gratifying activity for men as well as women, and must be given opportunities to develop confidence in their ability to provide such care via classes and practical, hands-on experiences (Klinman, 1986). Additionally, children need exposure to nurturant male teachers, especially during the elementary school years.

As the internal and external barriers to nurturant fathering are removed, men will be increasingly able to fill the void in their lives that stems from their lack of involvement in the care of their children. This development has the potential to be of enormous benefit to men, women, and the children that they jointly create.

REFERENCES

Abarbanel, A. (1979). Shared parenting after separation and divorce; A study of joint custody. *American Journal of Orthopsychiatry, 49*, 320–328.

Abelin, E. L. (1975). Some further observations and comments on the earliest role of the father. *International Journal of Psychoanalysis, 56*, 293–302.

Berg, B., & Rosenblum, N. (1977). Fathers in family therapy: A survey of family therapists. *Journal of Marriage and Family Counseling, 3*, 85–91.

Biller, H. B. (1982). Fatherhood: Implications for child and adult development. In B. B. Wolman (Ed.), *Handbook of developmental psychology.* Englewood Cliffs, NJ: Prentice-Hall.

Chodorow, N. (1978). *The reproduction of mothering: Psychoanalysis and the sociology of gender.* Berkeley: University of California Press.

Dinnerstein, D. (1976). *The mermaid and the minotaur: Sexual arrangements and human malaise.* New York: Harper & Row.

Fein, R. A. (1974). Men and young children. In J. Pleck & J. Sawyer (Eds.), *Men and masculinity.* Englewood Cliffs, NJ: Prentice-Hall.

Feldman, L. B. (1982). Sex roles and family dynamics. In F. Walsh (Ed.), *Normal family processes.* New York: Guilford.

Herman, J. L. (1981). *Father-daughter incest.* Cambridge, MA: Harvard University Press.

Hetherington, E. M., & Hagan, M. S. (1986). Divorced fathers: Stress, coping, and adjustment. In M. E. Lamb (Ed.), *The father's role: Applied perspectives.* New York: Wiley.

Heubeck, B., Detmering, J., & Russell, G. (1986). Father involvement and responsibility in family therapy. In M. E. Lamb (Ed.), *The father's role: Applied perspectives.* New York: Wiley.

Hodges, W. F. (1986). *Interventions for children of divorce: Custody, access, and psychotherapy.* New York: Wiley.

Hoffman, L. W. (1983). Increased fathering: effects on the mother. In M. E. Lamb & A. Sagi (Eds.), *Fatherhood and family policy.* Hillsdale, NJ: Erlbaum.

Jacobs, J. W. (1982). The effect of divorce on fathers: An overview of the literature. *American Journal of Psychiatry, 139*, 1235–1241.

Jacobs, J. W. (1983). Treatment of divorcing fathers: Social and psychotherapeutic considerations. *American Journal of Psychiatry, 140*, 1294–1299.

Klinman, D. G. (1986). Fathers and the educational system. In M. E. Lamb (Ed.), *The father's role: Applied perspectives.* New York: Wiley.

Kotelchuck, M. (1976). The infant's relationship to the father: Experimental evidence. In M. E. Lamb, (Ed.), *The role of the father in child development*. New York: Wiley.

Lamb, M. E. (Ed.). (1982). *Nontraditional families: Parenting and child development*. Hillsdale, NJ: L. Erlbaum.

Lamb, M. E., & Levine, J. A. (1983). The Swedish parental insurance policy: An experiment in social engineering. In M. E. Lamb and A. Sagi (Eds.), *Fatherhood and family policy*, Hillsdale, NJ: Erlbaum.

Levinson, D. J. (1978). *The seasons of a man's life*. New York: Ballantine.

Luepnitz, D. A. (1982). *Child custody: A study of families after divorce*. Lexington, MA: Lexington.

Mahler, M. S., Pine, F., & Bergman, A. (1975). *The psychological birth of the human infant*. New York: Basic Books.

Martin, D. H. (1985). Fathers and adolescents. In S. M. H. Hanson & F. W. Bozett (Eds.), *Dimensions of fatherhood*. Beverly Hills, CA: Sage.

McHale, S. M., & Huston, T. L. (1984). Men and women as parents: Sex role orientations, employment, and parental roles with infants. *Child Development, 55*, 1349–1361.

Parke, R. D., Hymel, S., Power, T. G., & Tinsley, B. R. (1980). Fathers and risk: A hospital-based model of intervention. In D. B. Sawin, R. C. Hawkins, L. O. Walker, & H. Penticuff (Eds.), *Psychosocial risks in infant-environment transactions*, New York: Brunner/Mazel.

Parke, R. D. (1981). *Fathers*. Cambridge, MA: Harvard University Press.

Parker, H., & Parker, S. (1986). Father–daughter sexual abuse: An emerging perspective. *American Journal of Orthopsychiatry, 56*, 531–549.

Pleck, J. H. (1979). Men's family work: Three perspectives and some new data. *The Family Coordinator, 28*, 481–488.

Pleck, J. H. (1986). Employment and fatherhood: Issues and innovative policies. In M. E. Lamb (Ed.), *The father's role: Applied perspectives*. New York: Wiley.

Pruett, K. D. (1987). *The nurturing father*. New York: Warner.

Radin, N. (1981). The role of the father in cognitive/academic intellectual development. In M. E. Lamb (Ed.) *The role of the father in child development* (2nd ed.). New York: Wiley.

Radin, N. (1982). Primary caregiving and role sharing fathers of preschoolers. In M. E. Lamb (Ed.), *Nontraditional families: Parenting and child development*. Hillsdale, NJ: Erlbaum.

Rosen, B., Jerdee, T. H., & Prestwich, T. L. (1975). Dual-career marital adjustment: Potential effects of discriminatory managerial attitudes. *Journal of Marriage and the Family, 37*, 565–572.

Rubin, L. B. (1983). *Intimate strangers: Men and women together*. New York: Harper & Row.

Russell, G. (1982). Shared-caregiving families: An Australian study. In

M. E. Lamb (Ed.), *Nontraditional families: Parenting and child development*. Hillsdale, NJ: Erlbaum.

Russell, G. (1986). Primary caretaking and role sharing fathers. In M. E. Lamb (Ed.), *The father's role: Applied perspectives*. New York: Wiley.

Russell, G., & Radin, N. (1983). Increased paternal participation: The father's perspective. In M. E. Lamb & A. Sagi (Eds.), *Fatherhood and family policy*. Hillsdale, NJ: Erlbaum.

Sagi, A. (1982). Antecedents and consequences of various degrees of paternal involvement in child rearing: The Israeli project. In M. E. Lamb (Ed.), *Nontraditional families*. Hillsdale, NJ: Erlbaum.

Santrock, J. W., & Warshak, R. A. (1986). Development, relationships, and legal/clinical considerations in father-custody families. In M. E. Lamb (Ed.), *The father's role: Applied perspectives*. New York: Wiley.

Santrock, J. W., Warshak, R. A., & Elliot, G. L. (1982). Social development and parent-child interaction in father-custody and stepmother families. In M. E. Lamb (Ed.), *Nontraditional families*. Hillsdale, NJ: Erlbaum.

Shapiro, R. J., & Budman, S. H. (1973). Defection, termination, and continuation in family and individual therapy. *Family Process, 12*, 55–67.

Steele, B. F. (1982). Abusive fathers. In S. Cath, A. Gurwitt, & J. M. Ross (Eds.), *Father and child: Developmental and clinical perspectives*. Boston: Little, Brown.

Steinman, S. (1981). The experience of children in a joint custody arrangement. *American Journal of Orthopsychiatry, 51*, 403–414.

Thorman, G. (1983). *Incestuous families*. Springfield, IL: Charles C. Thomas.

Tyler, A. H. (1986). The abusing father. In M. E. Lamb (Ed.), *The father's role: Applied perspectives*. New York: Wiley.

Vaillant, G. D. (1977). *Adaptations to life*. Boston: Little, Brown.

Watson, J. M. (1985). *Parental explanations of emotional disturbance and their relationship to the outcome of therapy*. Unpublished doctoral dissertation, Macquarie University, Sydney, Australia.

· 5 ·

Friendship between Men

ROBERT S. PASICK

A PERSONAL (HOPEFULLY HUMOROUS) PREFACE

In 1984 Richard Meth called me to collaborate with him and Larry Feldman on a presentation on men at the annual Orthopsychiatry meeting. I was to present the segment of the workshop on men and friendship. What follows is my account of what I learned while preparing for the workshop.

As an only child, friendship has always been particularly important to me. In fact, when I am frustrated or disappointed with friends, I feel that perhaps I place too much emphasis on friendship. So when I received a call three years ago from Richard Meth, asking me to give a talk on men and friendship at a professional conference, I accepted with a familiar blend of excitement and trepidation. As a clinical psychologist with a strong interest in gender issues, I knew immediately it was a good topic for me professionally; as someone with a high need for companionship, however, it would also be an emotionally charged subject.

I began my research on the topic at a large, familiar bookstore in town. I quickly found the women's studies section, which consisted of six long rows of books. I was unable to find the men's section nearby, but it was apparent that women had written extensively on gender. I finally asked an employee where I could find the men's section. He pointed to the stairs, until I explained I was not looking for the men's room. He laughed and gestured to the middle of the store.

All I could find was a section on sexuality. Again I asked for help, and was politely told to look lower. Sure enough, there was one shelf devoted to men, beneath shelves labeled "Homosexuality" and "Sexuality." As I started to peruse the handful of titles, I felt uncomfortable because I was standing in front of a rather prominent sign with "Homosexuality" written on it. I realized the trip had already provided two discoveries about men and friendship. First, women have devoted more energy than men to the study of gender relationships (at least they have written more books on the topic). Second, a major obstacle in friendships between men is men's discomfort with the topic of homosexuality.

I then decided merely reading more on the subject would be insufficient. My long dormant research voice told me it was time to do some serious inquiry into the topic. Oral research seemed most appropriate in the embryonic stage. It made sense to talk with male friends about friendship to give direction to a young project. I immediately thought of Rick, a good buddy from high school. But as I reached for the phone, it concerned me that Rick had not called me in a long time, and I had called him last. This surfaced a third point about friendship between men: most men keep score in their relationships, including contacts made and received. Like a structured game, if you made too many advances without reciprocation, the other person would be perceived as winning—which, of course, must be avoided at all costs.

For the sake of research, I swallowed my pride and picked up the phone. As it rang, it occurred to me that, despite being friends for 25 years, we had never actually talked about our friendship. Would he feel comfortable discussing it? I explained that I was preparing a presentation for work—which allowed us to talk freely about our friendship—and exposed a fourth truth: men can discuss virtually any topic if it can be connected to their jobs. Still, I was buoyed by the pleasant and productive conversation with my old friend.

My enthusiasm for learning more about men was understandably dampened the next morning, when I read an article in the newspaper which suggested that males may not serve any genetic purpose to the species. It seems that the conventional view that males are necessary for genetic variation is being challenged. Even more disheartening, Canadian scientists discovered that males appear to have no evolutionary function whatsoever. However, they did admit that males may be an effective mechanism for the contagious spread of parasitic DNA. I confess that I was reluctant to include this information in my list of male truths.

To further my research (or perhaps reaffirm my unscientific belief that males do count for something), I decided to expand my interviews with men about their friendships with men. However, because I was too awkward to call friends up for this express purpose, I arranged a game of poker at my house. I figured that I could accomplish two missions at once: I could observe men at play, like an anthropologist; and over pizza I could facilitate an informal talk about friendship, like a true psychologist (or maybe a TV talk show host).

It was clear after the first hand, however, that the game was not going to be as congenial as I had hoped. When the first dealer dealt a card out of turn, one player threw his cards down, upset that the hand was misdealt. The competitive, serious tone never abated the entire night, despite the fact that it was only penny ante and a case of beer was consumed. We teased and drank, but were a long way from a discussion of friendship. This event revealed a few more truths about friendships between men: when men get together, alcohol is almost always the lubricant used to facilitate more open discussion; though men may get together to socialize over an activity, the activity itself often eclipses the original intent of socializing; when men play a game, the rules are taken very seriously.

A couple days after the poker game, the National Collegiate basketball championship game aired, which provided another source of material for my presentation. I planned to videotape the commercials to examine how male friendships were portrayed on TV. A personal favorite features three men fishing and drinking beer, and closes with them around the campfire frying their catch, saying "It just doesn't get any better than this." Unfortunately, that commercial was not aired that night, nor were any that showed men relating to other men. Without exception, the ads presented men who could only relate to objects, including watches, sports cars, golf clubs, and financial portfolios. Another truth emerged: we are told that if a man owns the desired object, he also gets the desired woman. It is somewhat disappointing—even alarming—that friendship between men on TV is limited to grown men leaping on each other after a touchdown.

With my homework done, I headed off to the workshop in Chicago. The day went splendidly well, and the audience seemed to genuinely enjoy my presentation. When I climbed back on the shuttle bus to the airport, I felt tired but excited and satisfied. As I tend to do, I found myself listening to the conversation of two men sitting behind me. I was surprised to hear them talking about building forts for their children, placing their families ahead of their jobs, and even planning to spend more time together as friends. My curiosity had to be slaked, so I turned around, introduced myself and told them how wonderful it was to hear men talking about families and friendship instead of work. They responded warmly, and explained that they were ministers who had been in town for a conference on the urban poor. Another truth stood up to greet me: all men cannot be stamped as competitive, uncaring, and friendless. This feeling was reinforced when my wife met me at the door, congratulated me, and told me that another good male friend had called to see how the talk had gone.

WHERE HAVE ALL MY BUDDIES GONE?

Three years had passed since the presentation at the Orthopsychiatry Conference, when I began preparation for this chapter. This provided the opportunity to study the topic in greater depth, including investigating the current literature on male friendships, and talking with men in therapy, men's groups, and men's seminars. Despite this submersion, I still find the subject an enigma. Each time I think I have discovered a truth, contradicting evidence erodes my conviction.

There were, however, some definite patterns that emerged. Most men I talked to about friendship feel something is lacking, but have difficulty delineating exactly what that might be. To make matters more complicated, contradictions abound. For example, most men identify their wives or women partners as their best friends. Though they may be satisfied with this relationship, many are vaguely troubled that their best friend is not another man. Furthermore, many 30- to 50-year-old men long nostalgically for the type of close buddies they enjoyed in college or the service. They may consider a friend from that era as their best male friend, even though they have made little contact with this person since that time. Yet they cannot understand why they have not made any new male friends as close as the old ones. The 45-year-old protagonist of the film *Everybody's All-American* laments to his old college buddy: "Years ago I thought I'd go on making friends like you forever. But it hasn't happened . . . Why is that?"

Similarly, most husbands I talk to relish time spent with their male friends playing or going to sporting events—although they sense that this alone is not sufficient, especially compared to the more intimate friendships their wives have. Yet, however strongly these feelings may be, they still are unable to define precisely what is missing.

These experiences have made me wonder what it is men want from their friendships with men. Do we long for relationships (perpetuated by Hollywood and Madison Avenue) in which we are loyal and devoted, have glorious fun and freedom, and can also share our deepest, darkest secrets? The popularity of Butch Cassidy and the Sundance Kid, and Luke Skywalker and Han Solo might reflect this. Do men harbor a secret desire to be bound together in a common cause, as depicted in *The Dirty Dozen*?

Perhaps the illusions lie not only in our fantasies, but also the past. Were our boyhood friends really as close as we recall them, or do we allow sentiment to distort a bygone time, and believe too dearly in movies like *Stand By Me* and *American Grafitti*? We are reminded of the former star pitcher in Bruce Springsteen's *Glory Days* who cannot separate himself from his real and imagined past.

WHAT THE LITERATURE TELLS US

To read the current popular literature on friendships between men is to conclude that there is nothing redeeming about them. Clinical researchers give equally gloomy reports. McGill (1985), in a study of 700 men, found that most men "have no close friends," "do not value friendship highly," and finally, their "friendships are not as intimate as women's" (p. 157).

Another major researcher in the field, Levinson, reached similar conclusions in *The Seasons of a Man's Life* (1978).

> In our interviews, friendship was largely noticeable by its absence . . . Close friendship with a man or woman is rarely experienced by American men . . . A man may have a wide social network in which he has amicable, "friendly" relationships with many men and perhaps a few women. In general, however, most men do not have an intimate friend of the kind they recall fondly from boyhood or youth. We need to understand why friendship is so rare, and what consequences this deprivation has for adult life. (p. 335)

In *Intimate Strangers*, Rubin (1983) states that "women have more friendships (as distinct from collegial relationships or workmates) than men, and the difference in the content and quality of their friendships is marked and unmistakable" (p. 129).

Two social psychology researchers draw more encouraging conclusions from their analysis of male friendship. Sherrod (1987) reviewed the data compiled on this subject, and stressed that any study must recognize that men and women define friendships differently:

> . . . the meaning and content of male and female friendships are vastly different, on the whole: Men prefer activities over conversation, and men's conversations are far less intimate than women's conversations.
>
> According to the research, men seek not intimacy but companionship, not disclosure but commitment. Men's friendships involve unquestioned acceptance rather than unrestricted affirmation. (p. 220)

Mitchell (1986) also identified redeeming aspects of friendships between men in her study of 50 men and women between the ages of 30 and 40. She asked her subjects about their most important same-sex friendship, and found the most common pattern among men was a "competitive-accepting" relationship, in which friends enjoy both conversation and activities in their time together. Although competition was found to be a prominent aspect of this type of friendship, it was generally considered positive by the men in the study. Surprisingly, she also discovered that men were more satisfied with their friendships than women, whose relationships were categorized as "expressive-confirming" or "possessive-ambivalent." Both these patterns were described as more "open" than males', but also less satisfying. According to Mitchell (1986):

> The popular understanding was that if you were very competitive, you could not be intimate . . . Intimacy connotes a kind of vulnerability that was not associated with "being a man." One of the interesting things about the study is that there is a group of men who very clearly feel very intimate, close, vulnerable, and dependent upon their male friend—and who also feel competitive and masculine with that same male friend. (p. 53)

Such analyses help us understand the complex patterns in friendship between men. Men may not express "intimacy" as we commonly think of it in such activities as a racquet ball or poker game, yet competitive activities play a vital part in their well-being. They offer men comaraderie, pleasure, a sense of accomplishment, and an affirmation of masculinity. While men may not share feelings during these endeavors, they do enjoy each other's company. The appeal of these activities should not be underestimated; many men report that their tennis or softball game is the one event they most look forward to each week.

Two personal examples illustrate how important competitive activities can be for men. My father has bowled in the same league every Wednesday night since 1949, which has enabled him to maintain his friendships with boyhood and army male friends. During the evening he and his male friends share stories of their children, banter about their successes and failures, and, now, as they reach their 70s, complain of their aches and pains. Likewise, my father-in-law has played golf in the same foursome for 10 years. He considers the other three men close friends, though he rarely sees them away from the golf course. In the true spirit of friendship, he would be there for any of them if they ever needed help.

The pretense of these meetings is competition, yet the real pleasure that the men derive from these events comes from the opportunity to be with their friends. In their 70s, these men concern themselves less with who is the "best." Even when their performance is hampered by injury, they do not want to miss the weekly get-together because they so enjoy the company of their male friends. It is important to remember that such regular male-bonding activities provide an essential source of pleasure and support for men.

It is also true that not all men long for more intimacy with other men. Many are quite content to participate in activities where they may share joy and excitement, but never talk in depth about their personal lives. Many men view such relationships as true friendships.

Another consistent finding of the literature on male friendship is that most men consider their woman partner—their wife or girlfriend—their best friend. Men tend to believe women understand them better, and are easier to talk to about deeper concerns. This relationship strongly contrasts the one established with their male friends, whom they regard as buddies—someone to have a good time with, but not share serious problems. For this they depend on their women partners.

A CLINICAL PERSPECTIVE

To describe the difference between his friendship with his wife and his best male friend, a male client cited a time he felt particularly distressed over a major life crisis. When Lou talked to his wife about the problem, she listened carefully and thereafter inquired daily about his feelings on the matter. Lou also called a good friend with whom he played softball to talk about the situation. He acknowledged in therapy that calling had been a big risk. Over lunch his friend also listened, was supportive, and even offered some good advice. After the discussion ended, however, Lou's friend never followed up to ask how he had worked things out. Even at a party two months later, with ample opportunity to talk over the dilemma, this man never inquired about how Lou was feeling and how the crisis had been resolved.

Lou's disappointment with his friend had two effects. It reinforced his belief that his wife was his most reliable source of support, and it dampened any hope he had for developing an equally trusting relationship with another man. He was hurt by his friend's lack of concern, and eventually stopped pursuing the friendship. Such examples of men being let down by other men are all too common. Thus, it is hardly surprising that even those men in therapy who express their desire to expand their friendships from buddies to confidants are skeptical of the chances for success. Worse, they can rarely identify a friend of theirs who would be open to such a broadened relationship; even when they can, they are usually too afraid of rejection to take the initiative.

Lou's story represents one of the more perplexing aspects of friendship between men. Most men enjoy the comaraderie of their buddies, and the competitive-accepting pattern of friendship discussed earlier. Many, however, find this type of relationship insufficient by itself, and seek more closeness with their male friends—a special bond which they find missing in their adult lives. It is the kind of relationship Gottlieb (1983) described in a story in *The New York Times*, in which he recounts a reunion with his best male friends from college.

> Early one Friday morning last December, Hugh and I took off for Annapolis. The small plane flew not far from the ground, and we fell into silence watching the landscape below. Would our meeting with Charlie be simply a reliving of past associations, or would there be

more? Could we get beyond nostalgia for lost youth and move into a future friendship as well?

We arrived at the Baltimore–Washington airport, and, as we passed through the landing gate, there was Charlie looking for us. "Oh," I thought, drawing in my breath and my gut, "we are middle-aged for certain." Considerably heavier now, hair thinning, gray mixed with red, Charlie flashed us a familiar grin. We burst into excited shouts like small boys winning a Little League championship. We seized each other joyfully, jumping up and down, whooping, laughing, hugging and kissing. Arm in arm, we felt invincible, a reunited troika. We raced to the car, hopped in and drove off. Charlie was so excited telling us of his life over the past 15 years that we completely missed the highway turnoff and had to drive 30 miles out of the way before we came to Annapolis. His parents had both died, he explained. He had gambled everything on his second marriage, hoping it would give him the roots he sought, but, while he had two more children, it had not worked out. He was alone again.

We pulled up in front of the hotel where we were to stay. Hugh and I checked in and chose beds as college roommates do, flipping a coin for first choice. Charlie smiled. "'Hey, I bought us something." Three identical gift boxes containing three identical knitted ties, maroon with jaunty blue stripes. We laughed and put them on, three aging musketeers in the highest spirits despite the gray and drizzly day (p. 25).

Miller (1983) documents his search for new friendships with men in *Men and Friendship*. He kept a journal for several years to record the difficulty he experienced in his quest. At one moment, he laments, "despite what the new 'art of friendship' books say to the contrary, it is not easy to go out and make real friends after the age of thirty-five . . . above all else there is no natural matrix out of which friendship can easily arise and establish itself" (p. 55).

It is not only the lack of a natural forum that limits friendships between men, but also the strict adherence to the masculine code. In the next section we explore why adult men have difficulty establishing and maintaining the kind of intimate friendships with men that they recall from their youth.

RESTRICTED FRIENDSHIPS AND THE MASCULINE CODE

Why is it that even those men who recognize the limitations of their friendships with men, and desire to transcend the triviality of sports conversations over beer, find it so difficult to alter these patterns? What are the barriers that prevent men from developing and maintaining closer relationships with other men? We believe there are a number of factors responsible for this impasse: (1) men's adherence to a narrow definition of "masculinity"; (2) homophobia; (3) dependence on women for emotional support; (4) excessive devotion to work; (5) reluctance to face conflict; (6) unresolved relationships with fathers; and (7) the influence of advertising and the media. These will be addressed individually.

Adherence to a Narrow Definition of "Masculinity"

As discussed in Chapters 2 and 3, the masculine code emphasizes competition, autonomy, invulnerability, and power. These qualities run counter to the needs of meaningful friendships. Kohn (1986) demonstrates how competition can inhibit the development of satisfying personal relationships, in part because it is difficult to "switch from supportive to rivalrous and back again as if we were changing television stations" (p. 135). Kohn enumerates several reasons competition prevents closeness: in most contests the failure of one's opponents results in one's success, and is therefore desirable; competition runs counter to empathy, which is essential for healthy relationships; and competition can lead to envy, contempt, distrust, and, in its extreme forms, aggression. As boys, men were taught to view other boys as potential competitors, which rendered close friendship very difficult to sustain. We came to see friendship between men in win-lose terms.

Likewise, autonomy is not always conducive to closer friendships. Messages to "be your own man" establish a norm that results in men feeling weak if they have to rely on another. Our mythic heroes, such as Paul Bunyun, John Henry, the pioneer, and the cowboy, all faced challenges by themselves, fierce in their independence and strength. Even real idols who achieved their fame as part of a group are remembered and honored individually. Most boys know who Babe Ruth was, but few of his teammates who were integral to the Yankees success. Men seem to believe Lee Iacocca saved Chrysler single-handedly.

Because of the need to appear autonomous, invulnerable, and powerful, men experience internal conflict when they seek closer friendships with other men. Our male clients come to counseling in times of need, often the most acutely vulnerable points of their lives. Yet when we ask them if they have talked with a male friend about their problem, they almost always say no, stating that such a disclosure would humiliate them in front of their male friends. If men hide when they feel troubled, and only seek the company of other men when they are strong, how will their friendships expand?

Homophobia

As stated in Chapter 1, men's fear of homosexuality (or being perceived as homosexual) inhibits them from developing close friendships with men. This dread not only strictly limits the amount of touching men allow (mainly handshakes or on-the-field hugs), but also the variety of activities they enjoy together. One male client who did not like sports complained that he would feel awkward going out with another man for dinner or a movie. Because he lived in a small town, he feared other people might make inaccurate assumptions about his sexual preference if they saw him in these situations with a male friend. Even though he was not gay, nor believed he was prejudiced against gay men, he did not want others to gossip that he might be gay. He knew he would not risk this misconception if he and a friend went to a basketball game, a business lunch, or out for a couple beers, but dinner or a movie would not "look right."

We believe the extent of this anxiety is greatly underestimated. Homophobia is a major impetus behind the strict, traditional definition of masculine behavior most men follow. For many, any action that seems "unmanly" is equated with being a wimp, a sissy, or with homosexuality itself. Most men will avoid this association at tremendous cost, including the limitation or sacrifice of one's friendships. According to Miller (1983), most men confuse gender identity with sexual preference and effeminate behavior with homosexuality. "Part of the work every heterosexual man must perform to 'be a man' is never, ever, to make the slightest move that would cause himself or others to think his sexual preference in doubt" (p. 136).

Man's Best Friend Is a Woman

Our male clients usually maintained close male friends until they became seriously involved with a woman. Many 30- to 40-year-old men's best male friend was the first person they developed a strong relationship with, often in childhood, and almost always before they met their future spouse. We believe two factors contribute to this pattern. One, men's excessive devotion to work restricts greatly their opportunities to form new friendships. Second, as a man grows closer to the woman in his life, she often becomes his best friend. Like Lou, men come to rely on their women partners for support and intimacy, which diminishes their need for male friends. The fact that many men report feeling more comfortable with a woman is one explanation. They feel less need to hide their vulnerability with a woman, and feel that closeness is safer.

Some men feel abandoned when their friends wed. For example, Paul complained that "after Ken got married, I hardly saw him anymore. It was as if he had lost interest in me, and wanted to spend all his time with his wife." (Men's emotional dependence on women is explored further in Chapter 6).

Possessiveness is another facet of this problem. Men sometimes report that their wives do not respect their desire to spend more time with male friends, and attempt to restrict their "time out with the boys." A 17-year-old male client was upset because his girlfriend only permitted him one night per week with his friends. For men who are fathers with greater time constraints, this conflict between woman partners and male friends is more potent. Some husbands believe their wives are threatened by their male outings. Others consider their mates' wishes reasonable, in light of the already limited free time the men can offer. For these men, it is work first, family second, and themselves third, and any time left is for friends.

Excessive Devotion to Work

The most common reason men cite for their lack of friendships is insufficient time and energy, mainly due to the demands of their jobs. They would like to spend more time with friends, and most male clients regret the dearth of companions in their lives, yet they do not consider friendship a high priority. Working long hours is considered a badge of honor; wives and children require attention; and staying fit through exercise is considered important, especially in the media. But who ever hears any promotion of friendship? It is almost never claimed that friendship is vital to their career, family, prestige, or health (though the latter is being found to be true). Nor do many friends make demands to increase their time spent together.

Despite the genuine limitations time presents, it may only be a superficial reason for lack of friendships between men. A more plausible contributor may be the mind-set required by most work settings. On their jobs, men learn to be cautious about whom they trust, keep their problems to themselves, and compete for achievement. Although they may further one's career, these traits will hardly endear men to one another. They may respect a hard-nosed man at work, but will probably not share any private thoughts with him. This competitive ethos invades even their daily conversations, which one man described as "an ongoing pissing contest" (Pogrebin, 1987, p. 263).

Even when they are not working, men are ready to engage in competition with others. This can manifest itself in trying to impress with knowledge (knowing more about a current event), with success ("I am so busy with speaking engagements lately"), or even the progress of children ("Amy made the city swim team"). Many men respond to friends and acquaintances as they do to their competitors at work.

At work, men are also hesitant to place trust in others, lest they get taken advantage of. A men's therapy group I sponsor has shown me how difficult it is for men to trust each other with their feelings. They are only able to reveal private concerns after many months of prodding by the group leader. Still, the participants report sharing more with the group members than with their male friends. They consider revealing their feelings at work dangerous, because most work settings are too cut-throat. One male client, a supervisor, cited the difficulty he encountered when he befriended an employee and socialized with him outside of work. When the employee's performance slackened due to domestic problems, the supervisor faced the problem of firing a friend.

Reluctance to Face Conflict

Many male clients report that they tend to simply drop a relationship if it becomes too contentious, rather than work out the disagreement or grievance. The conflict need not be monumental to create a permanent schism between friends; it can be as minor as a humorous put-down delivered too harshly or the lack of reciprocation of an invitation. When we discuss friendships between men with our male clients, we are surprised at their tremendous sensitivity to personal slights, both real and imagined.

One male client took umbrage at a friend's teasing remarks. Rather than bringing the matter to his friend's attention, he decided to avoid this person altogether. At the therapist's urging he finally talked to his friend, who was surprisingly open to the criticism and apologized. The client asserted that he probably would never have been friendly with the man again had he not been encouraged to approach him. His reluctance to address the conflict springs from his difficulty in acknowledging pain—which he believed was tantamount to displaying weakness—and admitting that he cared enough about the relationship to be concerned about the incident.

His dilemma exposes the Catch-22 of friendships between men: to maintain a friendship, you must show concern for the other person; yet to do so might result in being perceived as sentimental, which is unmanly. If one is considered unmanly, what man will want to be his friend?

Unfinished Business with Fathers

The majority of adult male clients we see have unresolved relationships with their fathers. Either their fathers are viewed as authoritarian and threatening, or distant and uncaring. Most men are completely unable to talk with their fathers about their relationship (see Chapter 4). A father is, of course, the essential role model for most men. They tend to measure other men by the standards their fathers established. Such men's first instinct is to regard men they are unacquainted with either as potential threats, or as remote and not suitable for friendship.

Though difficulty with their fathers may make men wary of other men, it also creates an emotional vacuum they seek to fill with a paternal substitute. They frequently cultivate mentors at work, who are usually older and more experienced, to provide qualities their fathers lacked. They look to the mentors to be everything their fathers were not. Investing such status in the mentors can be problematic itself. Men often become as disillusioned with the mentors as they were with their fathers.

Influence of the Media

Most men watch sports events sponsored generously by beer companies, whose ads always show men drinking together at bars, golf courses, and fishing trips. (It is interesting to note that the men are almost always in large groups, suggesting that the beer companies suffer from an organizational homophobia, and are afraid to show two men talking together.) The men are rarely shown to be close friends—just drinking buddies, with few indications of intimacy.

Even the new television heroes, such as Bill Cosby, are close to their families and dedicated to their jobs, but spend almost no time with their friends. The model TV fathers on shows like "Father Knows Best," "Ozzie and Harriet," and "Leave It To Beaver" all considered their wives their best friends. TV fathers typically had one good buddy, to whom they could complain about their jobs, children, and wives. However, there was rarely any intimacy between such prototypical friends as Desi and Fred, Ralph Kramden and Ed Norton, or Ward Cleaver and Fred Rutherford. TV tends to reinforce male dependency on women for emotional connection. Even on fairly progressive shows like "Hill Street Blues," where the men do rely on each other at work, it is still the women to whom they reveal their feelings at the end of the day.

PRICE OF ISOLATION

In this section several obstacles to closer friendships between men are presented. Some may argue that this is just "much ado about nothing." So what if men do not have close friendships with each other? My answer is that the cost of these limitations for men and their families are monumental.

Dave, a 49-year-old male client, is typical of many men we see in our practice. He entered therapy due to the behavioral problems of his stepson. Dave graduated from a military academy and had numerous buddy relationships until he left the service to get married and took an accounting job in a large corporation. He had lost contact with most of his Navy friends, despite feeling that they had once developed close bonds. Since marrying, he just had not managed to find time to stay in touch with them, nor his three brothers, who lived 2,000 miles away. In the course of family therapy the acute differences that emerged between Dave and his wife eventually led to divorce. Throughout a bitter divorce battle, he had no one he felt he could turn to for support. Most of his married friends withdrew rather than taking sides, and he felt too ashamed and distant to call his old buddies.

During this period Dave was a member of a men's group, and he was able to vent his anger toward his wife in front of them. At times of greatest need, however, he would tend to miss the group sessions. He would only come when he could present a difficult situation that he had handled well, never during bouts of need or uncertainty. It always seemed essential that he conceal his vulnerability, even though other men in the group were also going through divorces and talking openly about them.

A few months after his separation, Dave developed a friendship with a woman who was going through a divorce. With her he could reveal his self-doubt and accept support. Somehow Dave felt that it was safer to talk with a woman than a man—though he recognized the emotional risk of starting a new intimate relationship with a woman before resolving the old one.

Like so many men, Dave camouflaged his absence of male friends. Because he was personable, well-liked, engaging, and seemingly confident, over the years he had had many buddies. In the Naval Academy he had learned to be "one of the boys" (though he admitted in therapy that he never felt completely comfortable with the "good old boy" role). As an officer he had enjoyed the perks of male privilege. He knew how to drink, play sports, chide, and compete. At a time when he ached for companionship and comfort, however, he found himself surprisingly distant from other men. Like most men who separate from their wives or girlfriends, Dave felt more comfortable turning to a woman than relying on his male buddies.

Dave's story illuminates many of the problems men face as a consequence of typical male friendship patterns. Although not readily apparent, men pay a high price for the restrictive nature of their friendships with men. A summary of the most common costs follows.

Without close friendships, men experience more stress.
Recent research by McAdams (1982) confirms that men who value and have a high need for intimacy report less stress and are more confident about the future than those who do not. McAdams (1982) also found that domestic troubles do not upset these men as much as those who value intimacy less; additionally, these men tend to have happier marriages.

House (1988) established that one's level of social connectedness is an important determinant of health and longevity. He notes that "social relationships, or the relative lack thereof, constitute a major risk factor for health—rivaling the side effect of well-established risk factors such as cigarette smoking, blood pressure, blood lipids, obesity and physical activity" (p. 541).

These findings seem to be particularly relevant for men. House (1988) states, "On balance men may benefit more from social relationships than women, especially in cross-gender relationships" (p. 542).

Dependence on wives or girlfriends for intimate friendships.
McAdams (1982) and House (1988) demonstrate how important close social relationships are for men, most of whom find this closeness with their opposite-sex significant other. This in itself may not present any troubles, but as clinicians we often see how this exclusivity can damage. With the increasing percentage of women going to work, women are less available to their husbands to fulfill the role of confidant. This absence can anger husbands and conjure feelings of resentment and jealousy. "While surveys show that almost two-thirds of men name their wives as their best friend," says Drury Sherrod, "only 40% of women return the complement" (Stains, 1986, p. 39).

When a wife is occupied with aging parents or illness, similar conflicts arise. New fathers also suffer their own form of postpartum depression, due to the temporary loss of their wives, who must care constantly for the newborn. Though he loves the baby and appreciates his wife for being such a good mother, the husband still misses his wife's attention.

During any type of family crisis, the wife often feels well-supported by her friends, while the husband may not receive similar sustenance from his friends. A male client discussed the conflicting feelings that arose when his son was admitted for emergency surgery. His wife wanted to spend each night of the 4-day stay at the hospital. The husband also wanted to stay, but his wife insisted that it was her responsibility alone. She received emotional support from several female friends who called during the stay (some of whom were wives of his friends). He felt isolated and scared. He was terribly worried about his son, yet neither his wife nor his friends lent him support. He felt guilty for being needy at a time of crisis, yet he could not deny his angst. He had expected to rely on his best friend—his wife—though he understood she was needed elsewhere.

Without close friends, men suffer alone.
When men do not share deep concerns with other men, they develop a distorted view of what is normal. If they do not reveal their vulnerabilities, disappointments, fears, and dreams to other men, they begin to believe that they are unique in having these feelings. By holding their cards close to their chest, men lose perspective and feel weak for experiencing feelings that other men apparently do not have. One client admitted he was anxious at work but felt he had no one he could talk with about it. Instead, he would wait until his wife was asleep and drink enough alcohol to put him to sleep. When the therapist assured him that his anxiety was justified given the demands of his job, it was a tremendous revelation for the client.

Those who participate in men's groups report that one of the greatest benefits of their participation is discovering that their self-doubt and sense of isolation are not unusual. This realization provides considerable relief, and enables them to face these difficult emotions with their dignity intact (see Chapter 11 for a more thorough discussion of men's groups).

Friends can sometimes be more objective than one's spouse in discussing a problem because they often do not have as high a stake in the outcome. A male friend might also better understand another man's predicament than a woman partner, as their situations are usually more analogous.

Without close friends, men are diminished as fathers.
If a man is not accustomed to close relationships with other men, he has more difficulty relating to his children, especially his sons. Without close friends, a man will not learn to be comfortable talking about himself or listening to others do so. This is particularly important when his children reach the teenage years, for he will be uneasy discussing adult issues and values with them, such as career choices, drugs, and sex. Instead, his contact with his children may be confined to sports and other competitive activities.

A generational cycle that perpetuates dysfunctionality may be set in motion if the father cannot develop close relationships with his sons. Greg was not close to his distant, critical, workaholic father. As an adult he was overly dependent on his wife and maintained no close male friends. With his sons the pattern repeated. He loved to play with them as infants, but as they reached adolescence Greg became demanding and withdrawn. Like his father he retreated into his work. Fortunately, he recognized the problem and entered therapy. Through participation in a men's group he learned to talk openly with other men and work through the pain he experienced with his father. Eventually he became a good friend to his sons.

CONCLUSION

Will male friendships increase in the next decade, or will men remain stuck in the same lonely patterns that have characterized men of the baby-boom generation? While creating this chapter, I was heartened by some encouraging signs of change in our culture.

- More men are joining men's groups with the expressed purpose of understanding themselves better and developing better male friendships.
- Movies like *The Big Chill, Everybody's All-American,* and *Stand By Me* all explore the issue of friendship between men and ask why such relationships are not more highly valued. These films reached a wide and enthusiastic audience.
- Public health programs are beginning to promote the benefits of social connectedness to our well-being. In California, a health campaign used the slogan, "Friends can be good medicine" (Stains, 1986, p. 37).
- During the 1988 professional basketball playoffs, the media focused on the close relationship between Isaiah Thomas and "Magic" Johnson, the two stars of the opposing teams. They kissed before the tip-off of each game, an unprecedented ritual.

Though these examples are encouraging, change in friendships between men will not come easily nor quickly. The obstacles discussed in this chapter are still present, and the risks for those who seek closer friendships are still great. A handy example is the aftermath of the Isaiah Thomas–Magic Johnson ritual. After publicly displaying their friendship, the two got into a shoving match later in the series. This incident prompted a lively discussion among those in my men's group, who debated the relative merits of closeness versus the need to be aggressive in competition. When virtually all other men are considered competitors, potential male friends are in short supply.

Yet there are plenty of men out there who desire more meaningful relationships with other men, though many will not outwardly admit this. I know this because I have met them; good friendships are available for men willing to take the chance. Those who have established such bonds will say that the potential benefits far outweigh whatever risks must be taken.

REFERENCES

Brod, H. (Ed.) (1987). *The making of masculinity*. Winchester, MA: Allen & Unwin.

Gottlieb, P. (1983, December 25). The Reunion. *The New York Times Magazine*, p. 25.

House, J. et al. (1988, July 2). Social relationships and health. *Science*, p. 541.

Kohn, A. (1986). *No contest*. Boston: Houghton Mifflin.

Levison, D. (1978). *The Seasons of a Man's Life*. New York: Ballantine.

McAdams, D. P. (1982). Sex and the TAT. *Journal of Personality Assessment, 52*, 379-409.

McGill, M. E. (1985). *The McGill report on male intimacy*. New York: Holt, Reinhart.

Miller, S. (1983). *Men and friendship*. Bath, England: Gateway Books.

Mitchell, C. (1986, April/May). The importance of friendship in adult lives. *Bostonia, 10*, pp. 52-54.

Pogrebin, L. C. (1987). *Among friends*. New York: McGraw-Hill.

Rubin, L. (1983). *Intimate strangers*. New York: Harper & Row.

Sherrod, D. (1987). The bonds of men. In H. Brod (Ed.), *The Making of Masculinities*. Winchester, MA: Allen and Unwin.

Stains, L. (1986, Spring). Men and friendship. *Men's Health*, p. 39.

PART II

MEN AND THE PROCESS OF CHANGE

·6·

Creating a Framework for Change

JO ANN ALLEN and SYLVIA GORDON

> I'm starting with the man in the mirror,
> I'm asking him to change his ways;
> And no message could have been any clearer,
> If you want to make the world a better place
> Take a look at yourself and then make a change.
> GLEN BALLARD

In spite of the fact that most men resist seeking help, we believe that they are increasingly finding their ways to the offices of therapists. Many are seeking help under duress, feeling forced to come by a significant other, an employer, or perhaps a physician. Perhaps the recent emphasis on involving families in treatment is partly responsible for the increase in male clients since therapists are more likely than in the past to insist that fathers and husbands participate in the meetings. Women who have been influenced by the Feminist Movement are more insistent that men share responsibilities for relationships. Consequently, their demands for changes often result in men entering therapy, sometimes under threat of separation. Employers are forcing men to seek help for addictions, and doctors are referring men for help with problems attributed to stress. Some men themselves, perhaps influenced by the media and significant people in their lives, are concerned that their priorities and beliefs are contributing to emotional, relationship, and physical problems. We read, with some regularity these days, about men dropping out of the corporate or professional world in order to devote themselves to relationships with their wives and children and to other pursuits.

131

Perhaps this trend toward therapy for men reflects a growing recognition that the "stronger sex" is the more "at-risk" sex in some important areas. Previous chapters of this book have amply demonstrated how the masculine values of independence, competitiveness, emotional control, and power may indeed be linked to a propensity for certain diseases and addictions and to a shortened life span. In addition, these same values are depriving many men of nurturing and satisfying relationships with families and friends, resulting in emotional isolation and depression.

The fact that more men are seeking help represents a challenge to therapists to find ways to make treatment not only palatable but effective for them. This chapter presents the concepts, ideas, and general methods that we have found useful in our clinical work with men. The following premises are the foundation of our framework:

1. Gender is a social construction and not a representation of an objective reality. The meanings attached to masculinity, such as rational thinking, control, and power, can be harmful and restrictive.
2. Many men want to and can change in ways to make their lives healthier, more satisfying, and longer.
3. A central issue to be addressed in helping men to change is their belief system about masculinity. Gender socialization contributes to stress, relationship difficulties, and health problems in men.
4. Therapy can help men develop insight and options, but it is necessary to consider issues of control, fear of dependency, and fear of vulnerability when engaging men in the therapeutic process. Therapists must be gender-sensitive and aware of their own biases if they are to work with men successfully.

PROBLEMS OF THE "MASCULINE MYSTIQUE"

There is a kind of "masculine mystique" made up of beliefs, values, and myths about masculinity. This mystique, which largely influences how many men behave and live their lives, is reflected to a great extent in the problems brought to the therapy room. The rigid behavior and limited perception involved in emphasizing control, independence, and competitiveness are emotionally restrictive and have harmful effects. Many men are victims of their own success in fulfilling these powerful messages about manhood.

One of the very real problems we are seeing with men revolves around the set of fears that are a tacit part of their socialization: fears of dependency, vulnerability, femininity, self-disclosure, and failure. One male client came to therapy while in the process of divorce experiencing extreme anxiety. He had never lived alone and had come face-to-face with his dependency upon women. To him, this realization meant that he was a failure, not so much as a husband, but as a man because he felt dependent and out of control. Experiencing feelings which he had been taught to fear as "unmanly" had generated enough stress to force him to seek help. Such fears, so threatening to the gender identity of most men, underlie many problems presented to therapists.

We find that these are confusing and unsettling times for most men. The Feminist Movement has forced changes in roles and relationships between the sexes. In addition, it has pushed men to consider the values of connectedness and interdependence—"women's values"—as a saner basis for living for both sexes (Surrey, 1978). Changes that challenge accepted "truths" are never easy; it is not surprising to find many men troubled and sometimes resentful. The traditional concepts of masculinity that they prize seem to be failing them.

In the confines of the therapy room, some men confess to feeling cheated out of a "birth right." As one man said, "I know I'm not supposed to feel this way but I just want to be an old-fashioned husband. I want to go to work and have a wife at home to take care of me." There is a resentment and a sadness that what was taught about the privileges of being a man and working hard do not accrue as readily in today's world. The problems and stresses that many men are experiencing revolve around these shifting images of masculinity especially in the areas of autonomy, emotionality, and relationships.

AUTONOMY AND "OUT-OF-BALANCE" LIVES

The developmental course for most men in our society is one that emphasizes separateness, independence, and control. Many of the problems presented to therapists by men have to do with the image of the mature male as the autonomous man who can "go it alone."

He must be invested in a job or career that leads to financial independence, which leads to power and control in societal institutions and/or in his family. From our observations of male clients, we have come to believe that this interpretation of autonomy is at the root of many problems experienced by men. Living up to the "masculine mystique" of the competitive and independent male is getting many men into emotional and physical trouble. Their lives are essentially out of balance.

"Out of balance" is a term we employ as an ecological metaphor for understanding some of the problems presented by clients. It seems particularly apt for describing the difficulties of men. The science of ecology has taught us that life-forms in the natural world constantly struggle to achieve and maintain an adaptive balance in which survival and growth are possible. We believe that human beings must also establish an adaptive balance with their physical and social environments in order to survive and to prosper. Interdependence provides the foundation for this kind of balance. Yet, the socialization of males stresses independence, separateness, and control rather than interdependence and connectedness.

The ecology of our lives provides texture and meaning. Women, out of necessity and out of the roles ascribed to them, have long valued connectedness, relatedness, and interdependence. They have known of the importance of relatedness to family, friends, religion, school, service providers, and cultural organizations as well as to work. Women have learned that it is critical to the well-being of their families and themselves to maintain such connections. On the other hand, males are routinely taught to deny their needs for connectedness and interdependence. This is particularly true in the realm of relationships. We believe that the necessity to deny such needs results in the inability to experience and to develop intimacy found in many men, which is often cited as a problem by their female partners.

Male clients often reveal, usually reluctantly, a deep longing for connectedness even though they have a sense of fear that accompanies this recognition. As one client, whose marriage was in jeopardy, said "I want to be able to feel close, but I don't know how except through sex. I've spent 50 years hiding my feelings. It's very uncomfortable trying to express feelings. I don't even know what they are half of the time."

Like the male client described above, many men hunger for close relationships with their spouses, their children, their parents, especially fathers, and their friends. Unfortunately, men have been socialized into the notion that relationships such as these should have a secondary priority to their real role in life, which is to succeed in the competitive realm of work. As a matter of fact, many men believe that relationships are the primary work of women and even come to depend upon women to take responsibility for maintaining connections with significant people in their lives. It is a common arrangement in marriages, and it is increasingly cited as a problem by women, that women are expected to maintain contact with extended family on both sides, and plan celebrations and social events with friends. This is one reason that men often feel so bereft and lonely when a marriage or relationship breaks up. They lose many more connections than just the relationship with the wife or woman lover.

Imbalance in connectedness, with an excessive amount of energy invested in one area with the consequent neglect of other essential interests, usually means that needs are going unmet. Stress and dysfunction are often the result. Typically, we have seen men experience the greatest imbalance between work and family. All too often men are overly invested in their work at the expense of familial relationships. These are not just high-powered, competitive business men or professional men who devote their lives to making a mark in their fields. Many blue-collar workers will take on a second job to escape the demands of close family involvement, and they do so with the blessing of society. Chapters 2 and 7 detail at length the work/ family imbalance, the economic and emotional dilemmas posed, and how therapy can be helpful.

RESTRICTED EMOTIONALITY, COMMUNICATION, AND RELATIONSHIP PROBLEMS

The "out-of-balance" metaphor extends into the internal life of men and results in an imbalance in the realm of feelings and emotions. Part of being "manly" is to deny and to dissociate from such natural human feelings as fear, sadness, and dependency. Logic and rational thought are valued as "masculine" traits, whereas so-called emotional responses, such as being fearful, compassionate, anxious, irrational, dependent, and indecisive, are designated as "feminine" characteristics and are thus to be avoided by men. The one emotion seemingly acceptable for men is anger, which, of course, leads to all sorts of problems. As the therapists who write other chapters of this section demonstrate, this restricted emotionality may well be associated with violence, addictive behavior, fear of intimacy, communication and relationship problems with women, and difficulty in parenting. We believe, as Eichler stated recently (1989), that one of the well-kept secrets in our society is that men suffer. Much of their suffering is unrecognized depression and fear, and, unfortunately, their suffering invades other lives.

One of the major ways the imbalance in the internal lives of many men is manifested is in communication problems with significant women in their lives. Satir, a leader in the family therapy field, writes of the necessity for congruence in healthy communication and relationships (1967). Congruence refers to a match between feeling and behavior. In other words, people who are congruent say what they mean and mean what they say. They recognize and "own" their feelings and express them comfortably and appropriately. The messages they send, both verbally and nonverbally, are clear and can be trusted. Both sexes are socialized to be incongruent since only certain feelings are appropriate for each gender. That is one reason why some men come across to women as distant, uncaring, unfeeling, inconsiderate, and even abusive. Women, on the other hand, often come across to men as irrational, demanding, overly emotional, and manipulative. It is little wonder that, "we can't communicate," is often stated as the major problem for couples. One of the tasks for couples' therapy is to work toward congruency in each individual in the couple so that feelings and needs can be communicated and responded to clearly.

MEN AND THERAPY

We do not believe therapy is the only answer to the problems facing men today. Certainly much of the change will, we hope, evolve in the larger society by redefining the meaning of masculinity and the roles of men. Therapy can, however, help develop personal solutions for those men who want to change, who feel at risk, or who have been mandated by the courts to change. Therapy with men is similar to that with women in some ways. It leads to self-understanding, and develops options for change and ways to change. However, therapy does offer most men opportunities they do not normally allow themselves, such as expressing their emotions, admitting to their emotional needs and confessing "weaknesses." It can help to educate them about the restrictiveness inherent in their beliefs about gender and develop options from a wide range of life-style choices.

Questions may be raised about how much of the therapy with men should be focused on gender issues. There are, of course, other issues and influences in the life of a man. Ethnicity, socioeconomic status, race, cultural heritage, family-of-origin, physical capabilities, and genetics all play a part in identity, resources, and problems of an individual male. Nevertheless, we think that gender socialization is a central concern and is a part of therapy that must be addressed with all male clients.

In much of our work with men, we draw upon notions of an "invented reality." This is taken from a theory, currently used widely by many family therapists, which holds that reality is not an external entity to be discovered but is something that we invent (Watzlawicz, 1984) and reinvent through language (Epstein & Loos, 1987). Shared "realities" become "truths" and are passed down by each generation in families, cultures, and societies. In this respect, gender meanings and gendered prescriptions for behavior are social constructions that fit a particular historical time frame (Hare-Mustin, 1988).

The idea of gender as a social construction is one that we have found immensely useful in helping men change their beliefs about masculinity. Using this kind of framework, we try to help male clients understand why they feel compelled to behave as they do even when such behavior is self-destructive. We believe that to help men with their problems, old "realities" must be replaced by new and more functional ideas about masculinity. In therapy we promote change in men by helping them to:

Understand the strong connection between their beliefs about gender and their problematic behaviors.

Change their "reality" about the meaning of masculinity to a more functional one.

Recognize their emotional needs and accept them as basic.

Understand their need for connectedness and find ways to connect.

Understand the influences of the family of origin on them and their beliefs and be able to differentiate themselves in healthy ways.

PROCESS OF THERAPY

There are several components that we draw upon in the process of helping men to understand themselves in terms of gender and to change in necessary ways. One component is psychoeducational, another involves facilitating the experiencing of long-denied feelings, and another has to do with furthering the emotional connections of men to significant and influential people in their (past and present) lives.

INVENTING A NEW REALITY: REDEFINING MASCULINITY

When we discover, as we do in most instances, that a client's beliefs about masculinity are part of his problem and stand in the way of change, we usually begin with an educational approach. Our goal is to help men change their beliefs about what it means to be male. If beliefs change, behavior is likely to follow suit. When men connect that central core of meanings and values with the problems that they are experiencing, it is more likely that new thoughts can replace old ones and result in more functional behavior patterns. In general, we start by assessing the beliefs of the individual client by:

Identifying the beliefs he holds about masculinity.
Identifying the sources of these beliefs in societal institutions and in the family of origin.
Identifying some of the potentially harmful results of these beliefs.
Connecting the beliefs to the presenting problems.
Emphasizing that these were not freely chosen beliefs, are not "carved in stone," and can be changed should he choose to do so.

From this kind of examination, many men begin to appreciate the restrictive quality of their belief system. Beginning with this kind of cognitive approach with men is generally helpful, and is received as nonthreatening and nonjudgmental, which is a considerable asset in getting men comfortable with the therapeutic process. As one male client in marital counseling explained, "I just can't get into the 'touchy-feely' stuff that my wife likes. Help me to think about what is wrong, and I bet I can change." Reframing his problems as a matter of a detrimental set of beliefs about the meaning of manhood was readily acceptable as an explanation for his relationship and communication difficulties. This "thinking through" process provided the impetus and direction for change, just as he had predicted.

A critical aspect of the psychoeducational beginning is to identify some of the negative effects of male socialization. We might, for example, discuss how men are taught to fear experiencing some basic human qualities such as vulnerability, dependency, and needs for nurturing. We go on to demonstrate that the vigilance against vulnerability can take its toll and become self-destructive. Our hope is that by exposing our male clients to some of the information about why men behave the way they do, we can begin to develop some new alternatives with them. Often, when men see how little choice they have had in generating their beliefs about masculinity, they react by questioning some of their lifelong premises and become able to imagine and accept different options.

Probably one of the most potentially disabling beliefs, and one we deal with frequently in therapy, has to do with autonomy. Early and later development of males stresses separation and differentiation. Feminist writers recently have made the point that autonomy and differentiation are aspects of connectedness, not opposing forces. One of the new realities we try to help men develop is contained in this quote: "There is no self without an other, and the challenge is to integrate autonomy and connection. One reason a man can look so enviably strong and separate is because women are playing out the other side for him" (Goodrich, 1988, p. 19). The challenge for the therapist is to help male clients to accept and be comfortable with the other side of his own self.

REDEFINING MASCULINITY: FAMILIES AND COUPLES

We strongly recommend including female partners and family members in at least some of the work around gender issues with men. They are certainly affected by his behavior and can contribute to his understanding its ramifications. In addition, these significant others are affected by any changes a man may experience in the process of therapy. There may be covert or overt resistance to change on the part of others with whom the male client is involved. Change falls within an interactional system.

Family members often have a way of inadvertently opening a window of opportunity for redefining masculinity. For example, one client was described by family members as "impossible to be close to." His wife and adult children complained that he was so independent he did not seem to need others. He was detached and unwilling to share anything about himself, though he constantly dispensed advice for their problems. They worried about his health and depression, but felt rejected if they tried to offer help. He finally explained, "I see no reason to talk about my concerns until I have worked out a solution. I'm supposed to be strong enough to take care of myself AND you." He revealed himself as someone who badly needed support, but harbored an overwhelming fear of being "weak" and "vulnerable." He rigidly clung to the belief that a man is the strength of his family and must be in charge.

In therapy, the family learned to respond to him by talking about how frightening and lonely it must be to constantly have to "look independent," especially when they were willing and able to support him without considering him "weak." The family was able to challenge him directly, to explain how these beliefs distanced him from them, and to tell him how much they missed him and the opportunity to give back to him. He gradually became able to reconsider the deeply ingrained and unquestioned habits of thought that separated him from his wife and children, and that prevented him from fulfilling his own needs. The definition of the problem was forever altered, and new solutions emerged.

The "invented reality" approach is also valuable in helping men understand their difficulties with the women in their lives. Problems often manifest as communication difficulties within couples. Many times, these difficulties are the result of two different communication "realities." Working with both partners presents an opportunity for them to redefine their communication problems as an outcome of two conflicting developmental realities. They can begin to appreciate how much their communication has to do with their preconceptions of how each gender is "supposed" to feel and behave. We have found that the source of many communication problems between men and women is their widely differing constructs of the nature of effective communication (Gilligan, 1982; Lerner, 1985).

Chapter 8, which is about working with men in couple relationships, deals extensively with communication problems. Basically, our work is guided by these considerations:

Many communication problems between the sexes are gender based.
Many men and women communicate through opposing perceptual
frames that limit the range of communication for both.

Therapy can help men and women construct a new communication "reality" in which congruency becomes possible.

HELPING MEN CONNECT:
OPENING UP EMOTIONAL LIFE

One of the next steps that we often find helpful and that flows directly
from the educative beginning is to get men in touch with their deep
sense of longing for connectedness. It is here that our notion of out-
of-balance lives can be a compelling idea. We can begin by demonstrating—even diagramming—how many men's lives are centered on
performance and competition in the work area. Discussion can then
focus on how, when work takes center stage, relationships are pushed
to the periphery. We often hear clients admit that relationships just
seem "to get in the way of work." They become a necessary nuisance
instead of a source of satisfaction and support. It is ironic that men
often end up losing, through overzealousness at work, those very
relationships that they had hoped to secure by hard work. Men connect
their ability to support a family and gain respect with achievement in
the workplace. In therapy, we stress that the solution becomes the
problem when this motivation overshadows other aspects of life. This
circumstance precludes the kind of connectedness to family, friends,
and other pursuits that could enrich and support a man. His life is out-
of-balance and out-of-control in many ways.

When we can successfully demonstrate that an out-of-balance life
is one likely to be full of stress and will sometimes lead to physical
and/or emotional difficulties, we can begin to open up the possibilities for developing a more adaptive balance or "goodness of fit"
(Germain and Gitterman, 1980). It is interesting how easily men can
relate to a reframing of a problem in this light. For example, one
man was referred to therapy by his doctor after an examination
revealed no physical source of his "heart pains" and accompanying
depression. In discussing this situation with him, it was clear to us
that his only meaningful connection was his job, which was unsatis-
fying, extremely competitive, and stressful. He felt exploited, yet
expended tremendous energy to get ahead in the company. He felt

trapped at work, with no apparent way out. Further, he had been granted custody of a 9-year-old son following a divorce 2 years previously. He was cut off from his family of origin and had few supportive relationships. He had neither the time nor the energy for friends, and he had never been able to make friends easily. The only adult relationship was with a woman who was pressuring him for a marriage for which he did not feel ready. He felt a great deal of anger, which he kept under strict control, and could not acknowledge the sadness and loneliness underneath the anger. The beginning of therapy helped him frame his depression as a deficit in emotional repertoire and support network. This would seem obvious, but, surprisingly, it was not, and it came as a relief to him to find that there was a sensible explanation for his problems.

One goal of our therapeutic approach is to help men understand interdependence and connectedness as positive values that anchor one's life. The adaptive balance is not achieved through passivity but is created through active choices made on the basis of developing self-knowledge, including an appreciation of present and past influences. We hope our male clients can embrace the notion that they need not be passive heirs to harmful legacies.

Therapy, in our view, can provide a setting in which a man can build a model of a balanced person, as one who can participate fully and comfortably in relationships without fear of compromising or losing autonomy or being overwhelmed by closeness. It is a setting in which we challenge the vision of maleness as logical and unemotional. We often introduce the idea that men may invoke "logic" because they fear experiencing strong emotions: An intellectual response can be a defense against normal, natural human feelings. Men can be helped to see the negative aftermath of their emotional denial. This kind of opening up can be done by working with men individually, in families, in couples, and/or in groups. The guideline for therapists is to make restrictive emotionality a treatment issue. If this can be done with some success, our male clients will have traveled a long way toward congruency in self, in communication, and in relationships.

CONNECTING WITH THE FAMILY OF ORIGIN

The key to unlocking change in a man often lies in helping him to gain an appreciation of the influence of his family of origin in ways he thinks and behaves. One of the most powerful and enduring influences in a man's life is the family in which he grew up. That is where he received his first training in what it means to be a man. In contrast, therefore, with Thomas Wolfe's dictum "You can't go home again," we believe it is often imperative for our male clients to go home, again and again. That journey can be the road to an understanding of themselves and to achieving the changes they seek. The following quote from Haverlick (1987) describes the reason for this.

> As is typical of many families, I was in an emotionally overclose relationship with my mother—one that was also overpositive—and in a more distant, intermittently conflictual, relationship with my father. There were many factors that contributed to the development and perpetuation of this pattern, including the large age gap between my father and me, the difference in levels of education, the recurring periods of competitiveness, my father's early periods of heavy drinking and the lack of shared or political philosophies. But it also had to do, as much, if not more, with patterns existing in the extended family: the generational patterns of mothers who are overpositive with respect to their sons while being more critical of their husbands; of fathers who never really experienced fathering themselves and who were led to believe that to be hard, tough, and strong was to be manly. For almost thirty-five years of my life, these patterns had been repeated time and time again, creating distance, distrust, anger, resentment and blame. (p. 305)

This quote details how the family of origin functions as the primary source of longing for connectedness present in many men. It also explains some of the emotional conflict that mitigates against men achieving connectedness.

For a variety of reasons, some cited above, sons can feel trapped "in the middle" between spouses who are distant from each other. They may experience guilt or disloyalty if they are close to either parent. In such a situation, it is not uncommon for a son to become guarded and angry with both his mother and his father. A chronic tension can develop between his desire for nurturing connected relationships with his parents and an urgency to pull away in the interests of self-protection. The experience described above is echoed in many of our clients' discussions of their families of origin. The result is often a learned disconnectedness, and a distrust and fear of intimacy.

Unresolved emotional issues rooted in the family of origin can impede the development of healthy and satisfying relationships throughout the life of a man. Unfortunately, ghosts from the past are not easily persuaded to disappear, and they continue to haunt a man's current relationships with his spouse, his children, his friends, and even his employers and co-workers. Emotions linked to the past, long denied and covered over, have a way of leaking out and contaminating the present, especially when a man is under stress. Perhaps that is the reason therapists hear men puzzle over finding themselves repeating behavior patterns that they detest in their parents. An unexamined past does have a way of repeating itself until it is understood. For example, therapists often hear a variation of the following, "I swore I would never treat my wife and kids the way my father did. Now I find I'm just like him in so many ways, and I can't seem to do anything about it."

Most therapists are familiar with the process and the procedures for involving clients in family of origin work. There is ample literature available for reference (e.g., Bowen, 1978; Kerr and Bowen, 1989; McGoldrick & Gerson, 1985). In addition, the following chapters provide numerous examples of therapy that is focused on family of origin issues. We want to underscore here that this approach, in combination with others already mentioned, is immensely valuable in helping men to rid themselves of emotional baggage around gender issues and relationships.

Much of the therapy around gender issues is devoted to helping men gain an appreciation of "where they came from" and an understanding of the tremendous influence of their families in their current lives. Through a thorough intergenerational search, they can understand how much their current "logical" choices were dictated by people from the past rather than being freely chosen. Men can also learn about the unresolved emotional issues from the past that trigger automatic behavioral responses in the present. Of great importance for many men is that they come to an acceptance of their need for connectedness, long buried with a deep sense of grief and often masked by feelings of anger and/or indifference.

Building on a growing understanding of familial influence, many men are able to interpret their current lives and relationships in a new light. As they identify the emotional triggers associated with earlier family relationships, they begin to see these triggers reappear—and reactivated—in other relationships. The development of such self-awareness is particularly useful in precipitating change in couple relationships. For example, one male client had learned to protect himself from his intrusive mother by staying busy with yardwork and other chores. His wife complained that he was a loner, particularly when any intense emotional situation would arise. He would often "hide" by taking care of the lawn or isolating himself in other ways at the slightest hint of intimacy or conflict. In therapy, he was able to clarify which issues belonged to the past and which were clearly associated with the couple relationship. He was able to realize how "triggers" from past experience were carrying over into the present, cutting him off from emotional support and satisfaction. Change came as he distinguished present relationships from harmful legacies and past patterns.

An important, perhaps crucial part of family of origin therapy is to help the client to gain an understanding of his parents as individuals. Chapters 10 and 11 will discuss this fully. Developing an intergenerational view of the family can often open the way to challenging beliefs and behavioral patterns. A man can perhaps then begin to see the unavailability of his father as the product of several generations of distancing fathers or perhaps as the product of cultural beliefs and messages. He may see the "guilt-tripping" of his mother as imbedded in generations of women whose only creative outlets were in family caretaking roles. He may for the first time become aware of the strength and caring of his parents, which his anger and guilt may have hidden from him. He can then make choices about how he wishes to relate to them now and which of their traits he wishes to emulate.

We believe that it is important, whenever possible, to help men to reconnect with their parents. Interestingly enough, in the process of reconnecting with parents as an adult, many men learn to reinterpret childhood events through the eyes of an adult. Without the egocentric focus of a child, a man can understand those events free from self-blame and negative interpretations. For example, one man, during a recent visit with his parents, reported observing the angry glances that his mother gave to his father as his father drank to the point of drunkenness. She did not openly express her feelings, but he noted that the anger on her face continued even as she turned to speak to him, her son. Often at those times, his mother would also hint that it was time for him to leave or would send him on some errand for her. The thought struck him with great impact that the anger that he always felt was directed at him in childhood was really meant for his father. He also realized that the many times when his mother seemed to be "trying to get rid of me" were probably her attempts to protect him from seeing his father drunk and out of control. He felt a great burden being lifted from him with the recognition that he had not been responsible for his mother's unhappiness, as he had thought as a child.

Working toward resolution of past conflicts and issues with parents is not a process of completely discarding the past. Change can involve the choice to maintain valued parts of the past and to give renewed meaning to the intergenerational heritage. Choice is the component that is freeing and growth-producing.

STARTING THERAPY WITH MEN

The remainder of this chapter is devoted to discussing the beginning of the process of therapy with male clients. Given their socialization, most men find it particularly painful to be in a position of needing help. It is critical, therefore, to start effectively if therapy is to progress well. It is especially important to consider the impact of the circumstances surrounding a man's entrance into therapy. Many therapists are now taking a much more egalitarian stance with all clients. They think of themselves as consultants to clients rather than experts who are in a "one-up" position. This works well and provides a comfortable beginning relationship. In addition, there are some effective joining techniques that are helpful with men.

Circumstances of the Referral

It is generally accepted among therapists that therapy is most effective when clients freely choose to engage in it. Their motivation is greater and they are more self-directed than those who enter involuntarily. It is our clinical observation that most male clients fall in the latter category, coerced by some external circumstance. This represents another psychological hurdle for both the male client and the therapist.

The more common external pressures that bring men to a therapist's office are discussed next.

Spouse

Though sometimes a spouse will request marital therapy to enhance an already healthy and committed relationship, most often the husband enters therapy only because his wife is urging change and/or threatening to leave. In some cases the wife is still very interested in saving the relationship, but in many cases by the time the husband finally agrees to therapy, the wife psychologically has moved on to other solutions. This leaves the man's shock and grief in the care of the therapist. Too often the situation resembles a recent case in which the workaholic husband finally agreed to marital counseling only to discover his wife was having an affair. Her emotional bags were packed to leave home as soon as the affair was uncovered in therapy.

Children

Often, a referral for therapy for the child or the child and family comes directly from the father and mother (the impetus usually provided by the latter) concerned over a depressed or acting-out child, or from school personnel who alert the parents. Our experience indicates that men are more comfortable entering therapy on behalf of their children than for any other reason, although they still bring a narrow problem-solving approach to therapy, not wanting to fully explore family dynamics. In a typical case, a child's petty theft was related to a broader family issue, discussion of which eventually led to marital counseling and divorce. The divorce ultimately relieved stress experienced, but not acknowledged, by everyone in the family.

Work

Men will enter therapy when they have lost their job or a promotion, or are unable to function effectively in their careers. The referral may come from an employment advisor, a friend, or an employer who wishes to retain an employee whose performance has deteriorated. Although there are numerous factors that can affect job performance, drug or alcohol abuse are often present in work-related referrals. Of course, positive change can occur as a result of crisis. For example, a middle-aged man who lost his executive-level job due to a company merger was able to use therapy both for support during his job search and later to examine his roles as husband, father, and son.

Court

An undeniably powerful source of pressure to enter therapy is a court order requiring this as part of a man's sentence for domestic violence,

sexual abuse, or drunk driving. Given the public and private humiliation of such mandated counseling, this referral is probably the least
likely to elicit commitment from the client; therapy under these
circumstances is often unsuccessful.

Doctor

The medical profession has become increasingly cognizant of the
psychological components of such physical diseases as hypertension,
ulcers, back problems, and heart disease. Many physicians will recommend counseling in addition to medication for these problems. However, as soon as the medical symptoms abate, the men will often cease
counseling.

Difficulties in Working with Men

Though no one enters therapy because their life is wonderful, it is
clear from the list above that most men start therapy because of some
external pressure, usually a crisis in the family, at work, or with
health. This crisis is frequently intensified by acute anxiety and/or
depression, often acknowledged by the client. Given this background,
the therapist may have little opportunity to gain the client's trust and
commitment to the therapeutic process. In the case of court-ordered
treatment, the client also brings considerable shame and hostility,
which are usually projected onto the therapist. Compounding all of
these factors is the male propensity for quick solutions; a tendency
that accelerates in crises.

To underscore the difficulty of working with men, one need only
contrast their circumstances of referral to those of women entering
therapy. Women rarely enter therapy for physical ailments or as a
result of court orders. Generally, men and women enter therapy for
the same kinds of reasons—the difference usually being the degree of
willingness, the stage of the problem, and who initiates the therapeutic process.

Because women are socialized to seek help for their problems, they
are generally quite comfortable entering therapy before a crisis forces
them to do so. They will often contact a therapist themselves, with
only the encouragement of a friend or a family member; men rarely
do this. Many of the obstacles men and their therapists face are not
present in the treatment of women.

Joining

Given the many impediments to engaging men in therapy, strategies must be employed that will reduce the inherent barriers. For example, emphasizing the release of feelings in the initial stages of therapy would turn off most male clients and reinforce their notion that therapy is a "touchy-feely" endeavor.

Therapists need to recognize and use the "male" model of communication to be effective with men, rather than the "female" model, which most therapy simulates. Especially at the outset of therapy, this requires therapists to concentrate on active strategies such as setting goals, using lists and diagrams, delineating tasks in sessions as well as "homework," and creating "contracts" to structure the therapeutic relationship. These approaches define the boundaries of therapy, and provide the male client some control over the process.

Perhaps the first point to address with men is the difficulty of entering therapy, and the courage it requires. The therapist should acknowledge that seeking help, discussing feelings, and participating in an ambiguous and open-ended relationship with a stranger are generally perceived as unmasculine activities and, therefore, can be threatening. Whatever reluctance and anxiety the client may harbor can then be regarded as appropriate to an alien situation. The therapist can then offer the client positive reinforcement for pursuing something so foreign to his socialization. Because most men consider seeking help to be an act of desperation and failure, reframing it as one of strength and determination helps the client feel in control of his self-doubts about beginning therapy.

A second—and an equally important—objective early in therapy is normalizing the man's immediate problem. Any man who is concerned about his children or his health, losing his job of his wife, or facing a jail sentence feels a tremendous sense of failure and loss of esteem. The therapist needs to help the client appreciate the larger context of his problem, allowing him to defuse some of his guilt and shame. It is less damaging to his ego to learn that his interpersonal style is primarily a result of family and societal conditions than to think it is due solely to his individual failures. This approach can be used with respect to the client's defense mechanisms developed in his family of origin, the limited number of role models he had, the variety of stresses in his life, and the effect of addictive substances on his judgment and actions. In this manner, the therapist helps the client recognize that he did the best he could. It is usually enormously relieving to discover that he is not stuck with a "defective" character and can unlearn many negative behaviors. The therapist can then explore with the client just how his coping strategies and limited relationship skills have contributed to his current problem(s).

A third component of the successful introduction to therapy flows from the one previously cited. Men carry the burden of "masculinity messages" such as being perfect, in control, and unemotional as part of their self-limiting defense mechanisms, and it is often very comforting for them to receive support for their struggles. Not only can such support reduce the sense of failure male clients feel, it can also heighten their self-respect. They can be taught to see that they recognized they needed assistance, and they sought it in spite of their resistance and anxiety. This is not an insignificant step, as most men persevere in their destructive paths rather than admit they need help. They may admit neediness to themselves, but withdraw from the problem by means of divorce, addiction, or suicide, rather than enter therapy.

The last point is especially relevant with men in couples' counseling. This strategy is even more psychoeducational than those mentioned previously as it presents some of the basic differences between the "masculine" and "feminine" models of the world. We find it fascinating that so few men and women have given serious consideration to the effect on their relationship of the woman's more affective and the man's more cognitive approaches to the world. Explaining that the differences in the mate they are trying to change are the result of socialization—not stubborness—is often eye-opening. Although there is some disappointment in learning they may never get from their spouse some of the responses they value from their same-sex friends, they can create a more solid and accepting relationship once they release the fantasies they have about one another.

CONCLUSION

This chapter has delineated the concepts and the ideas that provide the foundation for our treatment approach with men. Our view is a broad one, locating the sources of problems not only in the individual psyche and character, but in the interpersonal, familial, and societal environments from which men spring as human beings. We have set forth guidelines and treatment components on which we draw as we work with men individually, in families, as part of couples, and in groups. The chapters that follow will illustrate in some depth how to apply these ideas and methods to specific problem areas presented by men in therapy.

REFERENCES

Bowen, M. (1978). *Family therapy in clinical practice*. New York: Aronson.

Eichler, J. (1989). Presentation for Orthopsychiatry Annual Conference, New York City.

Epstein, E., & Loos, V. (1987). Some irreverant thoughts on the limits of family therapy. Paper presented at the Annual Conference for the American Association for Marriage and Family Therapy, Chicago, IL.

Gilligan, C. (1982). *In a different voice: Psychological theory and women's development*. Cambridge, MA: Harvard University Press.

Goodrich, T., Rampage, C., Ellman, B., & Halstead, K. (1988). *Feminist family therapy: A casebook* (p. 19). New York, London: Norton.

Hare-Mustin, R., & Maracek, J. (1988). The meaning of difference. *American Psychologist, 43*, 455–464.

Haverlick, J. J. (1987). A son's journey: Reflections after my father's death. In P. Titelman (Ed.), *The therapist's own family*. Northvale, NJ; London: Jason Aronson.

Kaplan, A. (1984). Female or male psychotherapists: New formulations. Stone Center for Developmental Services and Studies at Wellesley College. Work in progress.

Kaplan, A. (1979). Toward an analysis of sex-role related issues in the therapeutic relationship. *Psychiatry, 42*, 112–120.

Kerr, M., & Bowen, M. (1989). *Family evaluation*. New York: W. W. Norton.

Lerner, H. G. (1985). *The dance of anger*. New York: Harper & Row.

McGoldrick, M. & Gerson, R. (1985). *Genograms in family assessment*. New York: Norton.

Satir, V. (1967). *Conjoint family therapy*. Palo Alto, California: Basic Books.

Surrey, J. L. (1985). Self-in-relation: A theory of women's development. Some Center for Developmental Services and Studies at Wellesley College. Working paper.

Watzlawicz, P. (Ed.). (1984). *The invented reality: Contributions to constructivism*. New York: W. W. Norton.

·7·

Helping Men Understand Themselves

ROBERT S. PASICK, SYLVIA GORDON, and RICHARD L. METH

Oh yes I'm the great pretender,
Pretending that I'm doing well.
My need is such, I pretend too much,
I'm lonely, but no one can tell.
                    THE PLATTERS

For most men psychotherapy is the antithesis of "masculinity." To enter therapy a man must violate several tenets of the credo of "manhood." A "real man" is supposed to be self-reliant, invulnerable, and in control, whereas therapy requires the male client to admit he needs help, and to sacrifice some autonomy to the therapist. Because "real men" prefer rational, active solutions, therapy is viewed as a lot of emotional talk with little action. Further, the male preoccupation with knowing the rules and keeping score is seldom satisfied in therapy, which rarely provides such unambiguous data.

The very act of entering therapy clearly requires courage for most men, because it is an act that challenges the foundations of what is considered masculine. The most fundamental premise that the male client must reconsider is the notion that he is in complete control of himself and his surroundings.

In many ways Gene was typical of the first-time therapy client. Gene entered the therapist's office looking apprehensive and pressured, complaining he would not have been late if it were not for the heavy traffic and full parking lot. He admitted he had come to

152

therapy at his wife's urging, but he hoped it was not too late. Marcia, his wife of 18 years, had recently threatened to leave him and he could not understand why.

He worked hard all his life, and at age 50 he had finally become a financial success. This new-found wealth bought a lakeside house, two cars, a van, and a boat, though he said they did not have much time to use them. He and his wife went on wonderful trips each year (all scheduled around business matters). His job required him to be on the road 40% of the time, but at home he believed he was very devoted to his family. Gene admitted he used alcohol and tobacco in excess to relieve the pressures of his job. The fulcrum of his life was the American Dream: work hard and you can have it all. Despite the money and prestige, however, he faced the prospect of losing his wife, and wondered if he really had anything anymore.

As therapy began, Gene seemed guarded and uncertain. He said he wanted to reevaluate his life, and, as with every other challenge in his life, he felt confident that with enough effort, money, and the proper attitude, he would conquer this problem, too. "Doc, you tell me what needs to be done, and I'll do it. I don't want to lose my wife—without her, I'm nothing. I have no friends, just business acquaintances, and I can't talk to them. If she leaves, there's no one to take her place."

Despite Gene's claims that he badly wanted to participate in therapy, he was clearly uncomfortable and embarrassed to have to see a therapist. He admitted his wife had urged him for years to enter therapy, either with her or independently. Initially, he denied that any problem existed, and later argued that they could solve their problems without outside help. When his wife finally threatened to leave, however, Gene sought counseling.

Though he asked his therapist for advice, he was not comfortable hearing it. Gene was an executive more accustomed to giving orders than receiving them. The therapist was in a Catch-22: if he offered a suggestion Gene was resistant, but if he withheld advice, Gene perceived him to be indecisive or incompetent.

Perhaps most detrimental to the therapeutic process was Gene's outward confidence, which belied his underlying doubts and resentment. His professed faith in his ability to handle marital conflict as effectively as business problems concealed his deep fear that he might lose his wife and family.

This chapter explores the process of helping male clients like Gene understand themselves, including recognizing the obstacles to change. Three specific areas are addressed: men and emotions; masculinity, work, and money; and men and addictions.

MEN AND EMOTIONS

When we introduce the topic of "men and emotions," people inevitably have strong opinions. It is widely accepted in our society that men are not expected to discuss their feelings. Some people believe most men do not even experience intense feelings, except perhaps anger and lust. Others believe that men do harbor strong emotions, but tend to repress them. Proponents of this idea believe it is essential for men to get in touch with their feelings in order to resolve such problems as marital conflict and domestic violence.

From our clinical experience, we believe it is a myth that men have less capacity for feeling than women. We find men's feelings are just as intense and varied as those of women. What is true for men like Gene, however, is that they are not as adept as women at recognizing and expressing their feelings. This is not an innate difference, we believe, but rather a consequence of disparate gender socialization. As most boys grow to be men, they learn they should not openly express their feelings. The messages they receive include "big boys don't cry," "keep a stiff upper lip," and "keep your cool." Logical, rational behavior is regarded as "manly" by many, whereas being emotional is akin to "being sissy" for them. For these, composure is valued; if a boy is hurt, he learns not to cry. Likewise, if he is emotionally injured, he learns to conceal his vulnerability and disguise his needs.

The consequences of this mandate for men to repress feelings are monumental and of the utmost importance in the therapeutic process. The results of this mandate include the following:

1. *Decreased sensitivity to their feelings.* Because boys must not express their feelings, they learn to ignore, disguise, and detach themselves from their emotions. If a man does not feel, then he avoids the conflict of having to talk about it.

2. *Decreased sensitivity to the feelings of others.* Recognizing others' feelings requires empathy. Yet to be empathetic, men must acknowledge their own feelings, which may lead to internal conflict. Again, the easiest solution is for the man to ignore the feelings of

others. Gene, for example, was oblivious to his wife's unhappiness until she threatened to leave.

3. Intolerance or confusion by others' expression of feelings. Men learn to view such venting as a sign of weakness. Thus, boys who are expressive of their feelings are viewed as "sissies." Females are considered the "weaker sex" because they are so emotional. Gene learned to carefully guard his feelings.

4. The rational becomes too highly valued. Because rational thinking is perceived as the opposite of emotional behavior, many men believe they can suppress uncomfortable feelings if they are sufficiently rational. Popular magazines and mass-market self-help books coach people to not only be rational but also to think positively. Certainly, positive thinking is often beneficial, but it can also give men greater license to deny emotional states, which may be important to recognize. Gene's rational approach paid off handsomely at work, but was very ineffective at home.

5. Feelings are disguised. Men develop a variety of masks that serve as cover-ups for the direct expression of feeling. The roles of jokester and tease are two of the most common. When a man dares to reveal something important to him, he quickly follows the disclosure with a joke to make people laugh and reduce the intensity of his expression. The conflicting messages often confuse listeners, including the therapist, who may not know whether or not to take seriously such an expression. Humor is also used in intimate situations to dilute the strength of emotion men feel.

Another common mask is the macho personna. This requires the wearer to be fearless (even if he is afraid, he dare not show it), and to "never let things get to him" (he cannot let on that certain events can evoke emotions). A macho man never gets too attached to others, lest he develop strong feelings that would have to be acknowledged.

6. The avoidance of intimate, committed relationships. For many men getting close to someone means risking intense feelings toward that person. By retreating from commitment, they successfully avoid conflict over the expression of those feelings.

7. The use of addictive substances to avoid unpleasant feelings. Many men describe using alcohol or other drugs as a means to deaden their feelings. This need to numb feelings arises when they allow themselves no other outlet for the expression of these feelings. (This topic will be addressed more thoroughly later in this chapter.)

8. Men's emotional restrictiveness contributes to stress-related disorders. When men do not feel they can express their emotions, they have difficulty finding acceptable releases for their tension. Without an effective tension reducer, stress levels increase and can eventually lead to such problems as cardiovascular disease, ulcers, or chronic fatigue.

Bob, a 40-year-old accountant for a large firm, embodies many of these "rules." Married for the second time, he was a confessed workaholic who could not commit to vacation plans because "something might come up at the office." Under his professional demeanor he was surprisingly sensitive, yet he ignored his wife's tears in the sessions. When questioned about his behavior, he explained that he did not want to upset her by commenting on her anguish. Bob was very surprised to hear of his pained facial expression during his wife's crying.

At home, the more his wife tried to engage him in emotional discussions, the more Bob defended his position on intellectual grounds, or withdrew completely. He found it impossible to just listen to her recount her difficult day at work, and felt compelled to offer countless "solutions" and then became angry when she did not immediately respond.

Rules for Expressing Emotions

In the course of their development many boys are presented elaborate, often contradictory rules circumscribing the acceptable expression of feelings. As stated in Chapter 2, these guidelines have evolved to make men successful in the workplace, and many of these rules have been quite effective in promoting such achievement. In our practices, however, we often see that the same code that is so appropriate in the workplace fails miserably at home.

Our experience has shown that the first step for men trying to understand their emotions is recognizing the rules that govern their emotional expressiveness. Among the most common include the following:

1. Sports is an acceptable vehicle for expressing emotions. Because athletics are action-oriented, emotions can be discharged without verbalization, which makes them a popular form of expression for men. As players, men can participate enthusiastically without being emotionally exposed. The activity masks whatever feelings are aroused. Men can be close to other men without fearing the intimacy. Spectator sports enable men to vent a range of emotions in a publicly acceptable manner. They can cheer the triumphs, jeer the errors, worry about the outcome, and get angry with the officials and opponents. The playing field is one place where a man can comfortably and acceptably express disappointment over failure. Sports allow men to violate the otherwise strict code of male conduct.

2. *Men can depend on women to fulfill emotional needs.* As discussed in Chapter 3, many men learn that women will "take care of" their emotional needs. It is women with whom men can share their feelings. Men trust them to anticipate their needs, and respond accordingly.

3. *Sex is an appropriate outlet for men's emotions.* Men learn that during the sexual act they are free to express a spectrum of emotions even fuller than that expressed during sports. These emotions include love, tenderness, desire, and pleasure.

4. *Drinking alcohol enhances full expression.* Teenage boys quickly discover that the codes limiting emotional expressiveness are relaxed when males drink together. While drinking, they are permitted to display feelings considered taboo when sober, from joy to sadness to affection. It is not clear if it is the alcohol that reduces inhibitions, or whether it is the ritual itself that temporarily suspends the rules.

5. *The workplace is the least desirable place to express emotion.* Restricting emotions is crucial for men on the job, where any emotional display can jeopardize one's ascent in the corporate hierarchy. Most work settings reward those who are very composed and staid (see Chapter 2). Most male employees soon realize they must suppress their emotions at work, and not release them until they return home, if then.

6. *Men must handle upsetting experiences as quickly as possible.* Some events will occasionally penetrate the mental armor of even the most staunchly stoic man. A divorce or the death of someone close are two situations where it is considered appropriate to release deep feelings. However, despite the impact of such events, there is a strong need to absorb the pain quickly and "get on with one's life." It may be acceptable to experience grief for a few months, but persis-

tent distress will cause many men to question their masculine credentials. Consequently, men often fail to adequately grieve their losses, forcing them to suffer damaging side effects later in life.

John was a typical example of this last phenomenon. Devastated by his wife's affair and the break-up of their marriage, he sought out co-workers, relatives, and friends in order to express his anger and rage. John kept a journal and attended therapy regularly. He reported a reduced consumption of alcohol, cigarettes, and sports betting. This heightened expression of feelings lasted about 6 months, while the pain was most acute. He then began dating other women, and reported fewer and fewer of the meaningful dialogues he had shared with his support network. John also mentioned that he had resumed some social drinking, "under control," and began smoking a pipe, "not as bad as cigarettes." He stopped therapy soon after, feeling that he had healed his pain.

The rules for expressing emotions are not comprehensive or universally applicable, but are intended to provide the therapy with some valuable tools to help male clients discover the guidelines that they follow. As the male client becomes aware of his personal code of emotional conduct, the clinician may suggest that he monitor his ingrained rules as they surface between appointments. With the help of recent incidents, examining the client's personal views on emotion can be very illuminating.

Anger

Conventional wisdom holds that men are quick to anger. We are all too familiar with the popular movie genre in which men grit their teeth in rage, start fights, and bust up bars over slights both major and minor. Sports often reinforce this image of the hostile man. Managers kick dirt at umpires, tennis players scream obscenities, and hockey players swing sticks at each other.

Many men are referred to therapy because they have had difficulty controlling their anger at home. In our clinical practice, the male client's hostility hovers over many therapy sessions as an ever-present, yet often unspoken threat. In some cases, not only are the wife and children manipulated by the father's potential for outburst, but the therapist may also avoid sensitive issues lest they provoke the male client. Even when the expression of anger manifests itself in lesser forms of aggression, such as yelling, it still can be intimidating and affect the therapist's behavior.

Therefore, helping men understand and master their anger is a crucial aspect of therapy. It is often useful to approach this sensitive area by investigating with the client his early images of anger. An approach that has proven effective is exploring the client's family's attitudes towards anger. How did various family members vent anger, and how did the family respond to it? What situations were most likely to stir anger? After early experiences have been explored, questions about anger in the client's current family can be more safely approached. These questions often provide valuable comparisons.

From the conversations initiated by these questions, men can gain a different perspective on their anger. They may become aware of their own fear or sadness over anger in their family of origin. Talking about their past pain and sorrow can lead to a badly needed emotional release.

We have found it important to augment these questions with some basic facts about anger. From discussions with male clients we have discovered several recurring themes common to most clients: why anger is so common among men; the link between anger and aggressive behavior; and the fact that anger does not occur in a vacuum. These will be discussed in order.

Many boys learn to conceal their emotions and vulnerabilities, yet anger is often exempt from this rule. It may be considered a more "masculine" emotion because it appears strong and aggressive. Consequently, many of the feelings boys experience, such as jealousy and sadness, are channeled into anger. This pattern continues into adulthood. Further, many symbolic male heroes are permitted to get angry, and express this through aggression. It can be revealing to ask male clients who their boyhood heroes were, and why.

In addition, boys learn that "manhood" requires them to defend their beliefs. As the New Hampshire license plates admonish its citizens to "Live Free or Die," many men seem to believe it is crucial to "fight for what they believe is right." In therapy, we see many men who will not tolerate being treated in a manner that they perceive as unfair. For them "defending one's beliefs" is a license for unmitigated anger and aggressiveness if they feel they are being challenged.

Another reason anger becomes a predominant emotion for men is its effectiveness in maintaining family dominance. As stated earlier, being in control of situations is a premium for most males. A father's anger accomplishes this by instilling fear in his family. If therapists are to assist men in altering this pattern, we must help them challenge the assumption that they must be constantly in command. It is an extremely delicate issue for most male clients, and, if not handled sensitively, it can alienate them from therapy.

The concept of letting go of control can be helpful, and the Serenity Prayer has proven a useful model to men for learning this idea: "God grant me the serenity to accept the things I cannot change; the courage to change the things I can; and the wisdom to know the difference." Making a list of things the client must accept and those he can change can aid his perspective.

When discussing male anger we tend not to distinguish between anger—a feeling—and aggression, an action that includes yelling, name-calling, and striking objects and people. Obviously there is a crucial difference, and all men do not express their anger through aggression. In fact, some men fear expressing anger in any fashion. Yet the fear of anger turning into aggression lends anger much of its power.

It is important to teach men that it is possible and permissible to have angry feelings without performing aggressive acts. Anger can be discussed like any other feelings, and in fact it is quite desirable to do so. What is unacceptable, however, is transforming these feelings into hostility directed at family members.

In therapy it is essential for men to recognize and accept angry feelings as normal and inevitable. It is equally vital that they learn to express them verbally in a firm but calm manner. It is sufficient to say "the way you are behaving is angering me." Criticizing others' personalities, yelling, and name-calling are gratuitous and damaging methods of expression, and must be avoided.

This may seem an elementary distinction, but for many men discovering that they do not have to act on their anger is a crucial turning point in their lives. This is particularly important for men who were raised in abusive families, where no one was able to calmly discuss their feelings. Further, once a man learns to express anger in a civil manner, it is no longer necessary for him to suppress his angry feelings. Many men have developed an all-or-nothing response to anger: they either deny and restrain the feeling or explode in rage. The former method only increases the intensity of the inevitable outburst. By learning to express anger appropriately, they decrease the likelihood of regrettable explosions later.

Finally, we have found anger is usually a consequence of many contributing factors. To demonstrate this point, it is effective for the client to trace a sudden outburst to its antecedents. Most therapists readily recognize that our anger is often directed at things only remotely related to the original source of tension. For many men, however, this comes as a true revelation. Helping the client consider contributing factors of his anger can be accomplished by writing down the related events that occurred before the outburst.

In therapy Vince discussed an angry outburst toward his child for not putting away his scattered toys. By examining the day's events, we learned that Vince had been rebuked by his boss for lack of productivity. In the office his boss was dominant, and Vince's internal rules would not permit him to express any resentment over the unfair treatment. Vince stopped for a beer on the way home to help him "calm down," which may actually have decreased his tolerance. Arriving home, Vince noticed his lawn was uncut, and did not know when he would find the time to complete the chore with his busy schedule. Upon entering his house, he expected a warm greeting from his wife, who instead was on the phone. Yet it was not until Vince tripped over his 3-year-old son's fire truck that he finally snapped, yelling at him for being so sloppy.

In the discussion that followed, Vince and his wife were able to analyze the sequence of actions, and learn about his patterns of anger development. They discovered that Vince's anger is related to power struggles. At work Vince cannot express his anger at his boss. At home, however, he has considerable control over his son, who thus becomes a more acceptable outlet for his anger. They further realized Vince's anger builds over time, is magnified by alcohol, and does not release suddenly without antecedents. His pattern of anger is similar to his father's, who also became angry when he returned from work. Additionally, his dependence on his wife is unhealthy. If she is not available to talk with him about his feelings, he has no other outlet.

Clearly, however, these sobering findings easily suggested several positive conclusions. Vince was able to consider alternative courses of action, which enabled him to prevent hostile explosions in the future, and he could apologize to his son.

This method of sequence analysis has been effective in our work with men. Writing the sequence on a board enables the couple to analyze their actions without feeling judged. This approach is especially useful with couples who have violent arguments. It allows them to graphically examine the patterns that result in eruptions, and helps them focus on developing alternative patterns of action. Clearly, exploring the way men handle their emotions is a vital aspect of successful therapy.

Grief

Grief is another vital emotion to explore with men. We find that many of our clients as boys were not allowed to grieve at a time of loss, including the loss of a parent or even a pet or early love. Men have viewed grieving as something one should do quickly and privately, without prolonged or intense displays of emotion. Boys were often taught to keep "a stiff upper lip" in moments of loss. Many remember the powerful image of John F. Kennedy's young son, John, stoically saluting his father's casket.

Today, grief for men includes not only the loss of parents, but also the loss of the notion of a nurturing, mothering, self-sacrificing woman who will reward them for doing battle in the outside world by taking care of them at home. As a result of the Women's Movement, many men have lost what their fathers took for granted: the nurturing and undivided attention of their spouses. With the increased participation of women in the workplace, and the changes women have made in terms of greater independence, autonomy, and increased self-esteem, they are simply not as available to their husbands. This pattern of wives nurturing their husbands had become so familiar that we failed to recognize that men had become addicted to it. Consequently, as women's roles expanded, men have experienced withdrawal from that support.

This sense of loss may partially explain why men have been slow to change despite the progress of the Feminist Movement. Aggravating the situation is their inability to express or even recognize these feelings. As with any unacknowledged loss, the pain emerges indirectly, commonly through anger and withdrawal.

Such dependence and resulting grief can only be resolved by first acknowledging the problem, then proceeding with the difficult emotional task of expressing and overcoming the distress. Any efforts to induce change in men must take into account these critical underlying psychological factors. Persistent excoriations will only serve to engender resentment, not foster meaningful self-examination. Therapists know that one cannot change that which one is not willing to own up to. If men are to overcome their sense of loss around their spouses working, and the alterations women have made in their role expectations as wives, they must acknowledge the extent of their reliance on women for emotional support.

Although some men are able to confront their disappointment over the new order, most have simply denied the negative side effects. Some have indulged in addictive behaviors to mask their grief; others have avoided committment in their relationships. The high divorce rate of the 1980s clearly had many antecedents, but probably includes men's desire to look elsewhere for the nurturing they had grown up expecting in marriage.

It is not surprising that men who refuse to accept the changes in our society are often dissatisfied in their relationships. What is surprising, however, is the reaction men who try to alter their behavior receive from some women. As Miller (1988) observes, some women are not impressed with men who try to emulate their expressiveness, and are turned off by such "wimps." Therefore, some men not only have to sacrifice the devotion and status their fathers enjoyed, but are unable to replace them with new relationships and identities.

In addition to these considerable losses, many divorced fathers relinquish meaningful relationships with their children. This is partly a self-imposed punishment. Some divorced male clients admit the acute pain of separation recurs when they must return their children to their ex-wives after visitation. Because this is difficult for the men to face, they often end contact with their children. Robert De Niro's character in *Midnight Run* exemplified this type of father, who obviously had deep feelings for his daughter, yet had not seen her in 9 years and could not get close to her when he did.

To help men recover from these losses, they must become aware of their feelings. We believe, as Robert Bly, the poet, has suggested, that "grief, rather than anger, is the doorway to a man's feelings" (Miller, 1988, p. 54). To accomplish this, therapy can explore men's past losses or examine present ones to unearth men's sense of abandonment. Once identified, therapy can help men sort through their feelings to resolve old problems and understand the basis of their present ones.

Some men are surprisingly affected when they recall the painful separation from their mother as little boys. Unlike young girls, boys are taught that it is not only unacceptable to cling to their mothers, but that they must not cry over this separation. This is so ingrained in male clients that they are surprised to learn baby boys initially exhibit the same crying and clinging behavior as baby girls. This underscores the powerful impact of socialization on male clients.

Exposing the childhood pain men conceal from themselves and others helps them recognize the many other feelings they have learned to deny, including grief. In our practices we find that reopening these feelings produces awareness of other losses that were never sufficiently grieved, such as the loss of grandparents, friends, and pets. One male client's family moved frequently during his childhood. After thoroughly discussing the impact of this, he could acknowledge the considerable pain resulting from the repeated disruption of friendships and being the "new kid on the block." Once old feelings of loss are exhumed, the client can then see the importance of understanding and expressing these feeings in the present.

Another approach entails concentrating on the loneliness and isolation of the client's current life-style. Because many men are socialized to believe working and drinking excessively are expected of them, they are often unaware that these are actually learned patterns of denial. When they acknowledge their present emptiness, they often feel tremendous grief over the lack of fulfillment in their lives.

Tom entered therapy after the break-up of his live-in relationship. A successful engineer in his mid-30s, it soon became apparent that he had become both a workaholic and an alcoholic. Consequently, he was neither emotionally nor physically available for his partner. As he began to alter both of these addictive patterns, he felt extreme regret over the many squandered opportunities to acknowledge his and his partner's needs and feelings. This realization motivated him to establish a new relationship with his partner, and increase contact with his siblings, from whom he had become emotionally distant.

Exploring current grief as a means of gaining access to a lifetime of denied feelings is especially effective with divorced men. These men commonly did not realize how dependent they were on their wives to maintain their family connections until they were separated. It is usually the women who arrange family gatherings, send birthday cards, and respond to family emergencies. When divorced men assume these and other familial responsibilities, they often feel acutely inadequate. It is encouraging that when these men cease castigating themselves for not knowing what they never learned, they often work with considerable zeal and vigor at improving these relationships.

Another case demonstrates this pattern. Lou, in his mid-50s, was separated from his wife and stepson for several years. He evaded the grief of this relationship by not divorcing his wife and conducting several concurrent affairs with other women. Although some time was spent in therapy analyzing his current romantic relationships and his marriage, the greatest progress resulted from his efforts to renew his relationships with his mother and siblings. Lou was the eldest of three children, and had assumed a co-parent role after his father died when Lou was in his teens. He had never grieved the emotional unavailability of his mother after his father's death. He simply denied it and viewed his bereaved mother as another of the "kids" for whom he had to care. By exploring these issues in therapy and with his family members, he was finally able to grieve the nurturing he had not received and vent the burden of responsibility he had assumed at such a young age. This subsequently helped him recognize how he had reenacted some of these dynamics in his marriage and affairs. He also realized his unresolved marital status need not result in alienation from his stepson, with whom he soon spent a very pleasant week travelling.

MONEY, WORK, AND MASCULINITY

Our culture's concept of masculinity affects all aspects of a man's life, including his work, emotions, and sexuality. We believe a man must first recognize the pressures that our current models of masculinity impose before he can make significant changes in his life.

In order to discuss our male clients' conception of masculinity, we begin by asking, "What messages did you receive, while growing up, from family and friends about how you should behave as a man?" The most common responses include: "work hard," "keep your cool," "take risks," "don't let people take advantage of you," "don't let people see you cry," and "be financially successful." Each of these messages comes with a set of rules regulating how a man should feel and behave. Men need to realize that these rules direct many of their thoughts and actions, for better or worse.

To understand masculinity in American culture we must recognize the connections between power, money, and work. Few people would question that men in our society hold greater positions of occupational and political power than women. It is therefore interesting that in therapy many men say they do not feel they have any real power. Because many men work in a hierarchical structure, there is almost always someone who is above them on the company ladder, and therefore they tend to feel powerless.

Money

Although many men may not be able to precisely define "power," they are acutely aware of the symbols of power. In *Steps to an Ecology of Mind*, Bateson (1972) lists the most recognizable symbols of power: one's job; money; disregard for authority; sexual prowess; and gambling. Our clinical practices have found money to be the most potent of these symbols. A man's attitudes toward money will reveal much of his self-image as a man in our society; discussion of these attitudes may intiate a reevaluation of his preconceptions of masculinity.

Gene's case, discussed earlier, demonstrates the damaging effects of the blind ambition to earn more money. It can destroy a marriage, a family, and the male worker himself. Despite the overwhelming influence of money on the male psyche, surprisingly few therapists ask men about finances. It is as though money is the last taboo subject, and is viewed by therapists as impolite or even dangerous to discuss.

Surprisingly, however, in our practices we find that men are quite willing to discuss money. They are often relieved to do so, often because money requires more planning and creates more anxiety than anything else in their lives. To introduce the topic, it is usually sufficient to simply ask, "How much is enough?" Another effective strategy is to ask how a client's father viewed money, and how the client's views differ.

It is also important to determine how the male client feels about his income. How does he feel it compares with the income of his friends, father, and siblings? Does it satisfy his expectations? Where did his family stand financially? It is also interesting to note how comfortable the male client feels discussing money and with whom he feels comfortable doing so.

Once started, most men talk quite freely about money, and find it refreshing to do so. They are not only willing to discuss facts, but also their feelings about the subject. Pride and shame are often associated with money, in addition to anger, disappointment, and frustration.

How men spend their money can be as revealing as how they feel about their income. For many men the role of provider is so dominant that they can only express their love by purchasing gifts. Alternatives to this expression can be discussed by investigating how such gifts are received by family members. Many men are pleasantly surprised to learn that their loved ones prefer attention and time to material goods. It is a great relief to discover they need not work so hard to earn more money to win the affection of a child or spouse; they simply need to be with their family more.

Given the nature of male socialization in the United States, it is not surprising that work often dominates men's lives. As demonstrated in Chapter 2, a strong argument can be made that men are raised primarily to work. Being competitive, aware of the rules and the score, and concealing vulnerabilities are abilities that have traditionally been valuable in the workplace for men. When these skills are analyzed, however, it is clear they are maladaptive to other roles men must perform. A father's excessive competitiveness can be detrimental to a child's sense of well-being. Keeping score in a marital relationship prohibits cooperation and establishes an uneasy atmosphere. Burying fears inhibits men from developing close friendships with other men. The consequences of translating work habits to the home are clear.

Work

Despite the dominance of work in men's lives, many of our male clients are not fully aware of the extent of their absorption in their jobs. Like Gene, they may realize they spend many hours at work, but if asked to identify the highest priority in their lives, they usually say the family. They see work as a means to an end. They work hard to provide materially for their families, which they equate with being a good husband and father. Therefore it is easy for them to conclude that the harder they work, the more they will earn for their families, the better they will be perceived as husbands and fathers.

For the therapist, this pattern of thinking presents a real dilemma. The therapist may believe that the male client is working so strenuously he does not have enough time for his family or himself, and surmise that he is not behaving as a good father. Yet, the male client believes he is doing a good job precisely because he is spending so much time at work. Resolving this inconsistency provides a tough challenge for the therapist—especially for the male therapist who may also be struggling with the same conflict with his family.

In Chapter 2, we outlined some typical work-related problems men have and their causes. Clearly, this has little value unless we can use this knowledge to help our clients overcome their destructive habits. The following strategies have proven effective in therapy for men with work-related problems.

With a male client the clinician needs to devote a substantial portion of the assessment process to work issues: where he works; how much he works; whether or not he takes work home with him; and how he feels about his work situation. The male client's work history is also a valuable tool for analysis. What other jobs has he had? Is he doing what he has always wanted to do, or is his current job a compromise? Does he now wish to do something else? It is equally important to review the male client's relationships in the workplace. How well does he get along with his colleagues, his supervisors, and his subordinates?

In addition, we find it valuable to explore the work patterns of the male client's family. What did his father and mother do for a living? How well does he feel he has measured up to their expectations? Does he feel as successful as his siblings? Such questions can expose vital sources of conflict, which may manifest themselves in other facets of the male client's life.

The contemporary father must balance several demanding roles; thus, it is important to discover how the client handles them. Does he feel he spends too much time at work and not enough with his family? Poor health, and lack of exercise, rest, and good nutrition are prime indicators of excessive work habits.

Workaholic patterns are based not only on the number of hours actually worked, but also the extent to which work dominates the client's thoughts. Many clients find they cannot stop thinking about the office when they are away from it, and feel uncomfortable taking vacations. They may not have any interests or friends outside of work, and have difficulty imagining retirement. Workaholics also tend to indulge in severe self-criticism when something goes wrong on the job. Many work settings reinforce the patterns described here, which often contribute to problems with spouses, children, and friends. All these aspects of workaholism can be fruitful to explore with male clients. The following questions are useful in assessing the extent of the client's absorption with his job:

1. Can you always justify working more?
2. Do you feel lost without work to do?
3. Are your friends, spouse or children concerned that you work too much?
4. Do you worry that you work too much?
5. Can you exercise control over the amount of work you do for an extended period of time?
6. Do you hide from your problems by working more?
7. Do you boast of your exploits at work?
8. Can you imagine living without work? How much would you work if you didn't need the money?
9. Do you feel you have a choice over how much you work?
10. Do you lie about how much you work?

The issues presented above can open discussions about work that lead to meaningful change for many clients. Whether it is individual, marital, family, or group therapy, such conversations serve as catalysts to reassess the role of work in their lives. For others, however, this will not generate sufficient motivation for real improvement. The obstacles for these men are great. They are often extremely resistant to the very suggestion that they alter their work patterns. Work is often the one area of their lives where they truly feel good about themselves. They often work for organizations that require excessive work habits; job security and benefit packages often prohibit men from leaving unsatisfactory jobs. Many men, even those who earn large salaries, spend so much and have such heavy debts that they depend on their jobs to pay off loans and maintain their elaborate life-styles.

Guidelines

The motivations for such work habits may be plausible or not, but the point is clear: Such men must realize their work situation is harmful to their families and themselves. We offer therapists the following suggestions to help these men:

1. A psychoeducational approach is effective for demonstrating how men have been raised to work. (Much of the material in Chapter 2 can be discussed with men or couples.) Specific questions should be asked to determine how valid the client feels this concept is in his own life. It is also important for the therapist to present the inherent risks of workaholism and success addiction.

2. It is often useful for the therapist to have men (or couples) write down their goals for balancing their work and home life. Do they have definite ideas of how much time should be devoted to work? Do financial goals comply with work patterns? Then have them list and rank the obstacles to change according to their level of difficulty, and brainstorm solutions for each. In this manner, impediments are transformed into steps toward change.

3. It is important for men to set non-work-related goals. If they are to reduce the importance of work in their lives, they must learn to increase the value of family, play, and socializing.

4. Male clients should also examine their relationships with other men. Do they have friends outside of work? Do they talk to their friends about things unrelated to their jobs, including their doubts, joys, and personal goals? If not, they need encouragement to do so. In some cases a men's support group can be very helpful.

5. Men should also be urged to apply their work skills to the home. For example, if they are creative at work, they can learn to be creative at home, or apply their organizational skills to the kitchen. They need to perceive of learning new skills at home as an invigorating experience.

6. In many couples the woman treats the man at home as her assistant, which men often resent. Men are often better able to make the transition from work to home if they have full responsibility for certain tasks, or for certain times of the day or week. This may require the wife to relax her standards somewhat or accept new ways of having the chores completed, but the result is often a healthier home situation. The man also needs to more readily accept the role of "student" when it comes to learning how to do "housework" and "parenting."

7. Because few men have been taught how to take care of children, they may need a lot of support to become adept at child care. If a husband is to make worthwhile contributions to the home, generous doses of support and information from the therapist are essential.

8. Most important, men must be encouraged to believe they can change their work patterns. They have been so powerfully condi-

tioned to perceive work as their primary role that many men do not believe such fundamental changes are possible. It is crucial for the therapist to be sensitive to the fact that the work ethic is firmly ingrained in the male psyche. Altering patterns of work requires the therapist's patience and understanding, as well as the courage, trust, and conviction of the male client.

Masculinity

A man is able to make significant changes when he begins to recognize the limitations and potential destructiveness of the traditional male role. Men need to understand what it means to them to grow up male in their particular culture. It is obviously not just a biological phenomenon, nor is it completed with the end of puberty, nor graduation from high school. Being a man is a concept taught to boys from the time they learn to talk, if not sooner. Males learn to evaluate their actions according to their own criteria of "acting like a man." Exactly what this means varies greatly across all kinds of groups, but in therapy it is important to determine what "being a man" means to each client.

To further help men understand how they are still influenced by society's concept of masculinity, a number of approaches have proven useful, including how the messages the client received from his family about masculinity differed from those given by the neighborhood kids. Many male clients were told by their parents to "be good boys," whereas their peers often challenged them to experiment with risky behavior. They feared that if they did not "take the dare," they exposed themselves to being thought of as "unmanly." Here are some approaches to sorting out a male client's perception of masculinity:

• Ask how his father's messages differed from those of his mother, and how he sorted these out. The father's advice was often considered the more reliable guide to manhood, though it was usually the mother who kept abreast of the boy's daily activities. What conflicts resulted from trying to follow both parents' expectations?

• How did his expectations of manhood change over time? This is intended to encourage men to consider the developmental aspects of manhood, which naturally become more pronounced as they enter adolescence.

• What messages did he receive about how men are to relate to women and other men? This is especially valuable for those whose marriages are struggling, or for those who have few close friendships with men.

• Which messages about manhood does he believe in, and which does he now reject? This will help men see how their beliefs have changed since adolescence. Which have been the most helpful, and most detrimental? Which ones does he want to pass on to his children? This process heightens the awareness that enables men to change.

• Discussing contemporary news or sports events can reveal the client's view of masculinity in an unthreatening manner. For example, what did he think about the Ivan Boesky Wall Street scandal? Could he relate to the extreme pressures on Boesky to earn money? If the therapist is a sports fan, current sports events provide rich examples of the notion of masculinity in our society. One therapist talked with a client about the need to "never let another man get the best of you." The example used was an incident in a hockey game in which one player took a vicious swing at another to get even for a body check he received earlier. By presenting this event, they were able to freely discuss the concept of male competition, which led to a conversation about the client's highly stressful work environment.

• Analyzing advertisements can also prompt male clients to consider the messages they still receive about contemporary masculinity. It is useful to ask the client what expectations are expressed through radio, TV, and print media. Often they are surprised at how inaccurately men are portrayed. The men in ads are either drinking with their friends, on an adventure, or driving a car with a beautiful young woman. According to such ads, life's objective is to earn enough money to buy the sporty car, which will enable the man to "win the woman."

• TV shows are also fertile ground for examining our culture's expectations of manhood. They tend to portray men either as superheroes who never experience fear, defeat, or mundane commitments like wives and children (e.g., Tom Selleck on "Magnum P.I."); or else they are portrayed as ineffectual, obnoxious men who are constantly outwitted by their manipulative wives (e.g., "The Jeffersons"). Even "The Cosby Show" often casts Cliff as dependent on his wife to control his impulses to overwork and overeat. Interestingly, this show is one of the most provocative to discuss with male clients, because some feel he is a hero and others a threat to their conception of manhood.

• Partly due to VCRs, Hollywood's depictions of men have become another accessible source of investigation. As in TV, many of the contemporary male heroes in movies present models that are often superficial, narrow, sexist, and impossible to emulate. For example, in "Beverly Hills Cop," Eddie Murphy's character, Axel Foley, is a danger-seeking renegade police officer who manages to outsmart, outtalk, and outswear everyone he encounters. This character reinforces several myths of male expectations: men must be resourceful enough to get out of any jam; they cannot allow themselves to be controlled by others; they attract women with their toughness and profanity, and are supposed to treat them as sex objects; and bullets will not kill those who are in the right. Movies offer mixed messages about fathering. In *Kramer Versus Kramer*, Dustin Hoffman played a sensitive, caring, and involved father. One of the more powerful moments of the movie occurred when a doctor asks the father to wait outside while he stitched up his son. Hoffman replies, "He's my son, and I will stay right here where he needs me." Many men we see have also commented on the recent film *Three Men and a Baby*, which gains much of its humor by poking fun at men's ignorance of raising children. A number of clients felt this movie reinforced the notion that men should stick to making money and stay away from diapers. Obviously, such films do little to show the gratifying qualities of fatherhood.

• Another effective exercise is to ask men to name contemporary movie stars who do not fit the macho stereotype. Most men can identify some of these actors, such as Woody Allen and Charles Grodin, but they usually express ambivalence toward such role models. Even the most "liberated" men seem to prefer movies with Clint Eastwood or Sylvester Stallone, who present themselves as supermasculine warriors impervious to any pain or vulnerability. Asking men what movies they enjoy can provide valuable insights into how a man thinks and feels about himself.

It was stated earlier that men have a tendency to measure themselves against other men, and this competitiveness may develop from a young age. Keeping score, comparing oneself to others, and scrutinizing one's place in the hierarchy are all important concepts to address in determining how a male client perceives himself. Such discussions often elicit strong reactions from male clients, including sharp memories of one's standing while growing up, and as an adult.

The therapist can also ask the male client how he compared himself to other boys growing up. Was he athletic? Did he consider himself strong or weak? Where did he stand academically in school? An equally relevant issue is the introduction of girls in his life. How did he compare to other boys when he became interested in girls? Did he have as many dates as his friends? Were girls as interested in him as other boys? Was he shy or confident? Did he feel attractive or not? What were his images of a successful teenager? How did he compare to that image? Questions that require the male client to compare himself to other men are more likely to begin a lively discussion than those that only ask for his individual feelings.

Despite the present insignificance of events so far in the past, the feelings men still attach to boyhood status are hardly trivial. One client recalled how painful it was to bat last in little league baseball. In fact, when he came to therapy he was still trying to resolve the emotional trauma of boyhood by pushing himself at work. He was doing everything possible to become the vice president of a division he described as "very competitive and cut-throat." Oblivious to the costs for him and his family, the consequences were ignored until a routine physical examination revealed an alarmingly high blood pressure.

Another client, a 24-year-old man, felt very anxious on his new job. In searching for the source of his insecurity the therapist asked him how he compared to his adolescent peers. He reported that he was a poor athlete, and his self-esteem was battered by the teasing he received because he could not catch a ball. The ridicule made him angry, and prompted him to withdraw from other boys. Asking him to compare himself to his peers showed him the influence of his peers and the stereotypical male role as important sources of conflict in his life. Uncovering his dormant feelings from adolescence freed him to explore his current feelings in greater depth.

MEN AND ADDICTIONS

In our culture masculinity and addictions are inextricably linked; the combination is so prevalent and devastating that therapists should not ignore it. The connections between illness and alcoholism, and substance abuse and violent crime (including sexual assault and child abuse) have been clearly established. Cocaine addiction is destroying young people directly through overdose and drug wars, and indirectly through decimated neighborhoods and lost ambition. Sexual addiction is not only harmful for the addict, it can lead to the psychological and physical degradation of women. Likewise, workaholism denies the workaholics full and balanced lives while also removing them from their families.

These addictions strip their victims of their self-esteem. Addicts question their self-control and misjudge their strength. Every addiction prompts the male addict to retreat into denial to himself and his family. Such an environment is ripe to spawn more addictions in future generations.

Role of Therapy

The prevalence of addictive patterns in our male clients is often directly linked to male gender-role conditioning. Both the etiology of addictive behavior and its remarkable obstinacy have their antecedents in the method of raising males in American society. To help men confront and free themselves from addictive patterns, it is important to review the various ways addictive patterns are developed and sustained by male gender-role conditioning.

The initial contact with the addictive substance is often associated with a desire to be "a real man." In the most common addictions—to alcohol and smoking—this link is bolstered by advertising. A recent study of beer ads reported in *Sports Illustrated* (Johnson, 1988) demonstrated how beer commercials inform our male youth that "real men" (especially those whose work is physical) drink beer as a reward for a hard day's work. Such commercials associate beer with fast cars, beautiful women, male comaraderie, and tests of manhood. Similarly, cigarette ads present men almost exclusively in "real men" roles, such as cowboys, race car drivers, and construction workers. Therefore, being a "real man" is not only linked to alcohol and cigarettes, but also to danger.

It is this need to take risks that also allows men to discount the hazards of addictive substances. In fact, some men become addicted to substances precisely because they represent risk, particularly young men who are seeking opportunities to validate their masculinity. Thus, because the drug prevention ads warn of the real dangers of these substances, they can unwittingly have a paradoxical effect on the male audience.

The objects of addiction are also appealing because they artificially enhance a man's sense of mastery. Excessive alcohol, drugs, work patterns, and sexual habits can all buttress the male ego. By drinking, a shy man at a party can temporarily be outgoing. However, his motor and cognitive abilities decline at the same time his boldness soars.

By presenting an acceptable outlet for emotional behavior, addictions allow men to more comfortably maintain their emotional restrictiveness at other times. Most of the substances or processes to which men become addicted have a "feel good" quality to them. They usually provide an intensely emotional experience for men who otherwise take great pains to limit such moments. Consistently getting high or having multiple sexual experiences feels emotionally expansive to someone who might otherwise feel emotionally inhibited.

Addictions are often associated with male bonding. Male socialization dictates that men must not get too close to each other, unless they are drinking, taking drugs, or gambling. Men drink in neighborhood bars or at sporting events. Cocaine and marijuana are generally used at parties, where men are together in groups. Men gamble at a card table or race track. Men thus learn to associate friendship with addictions. A common refrain for male friends is "let's get together for a beer or two." It is not surprising that addictive substances become part of the fabric of male bonding. A major obstacle to overcoming addictions is the fear of being cut off from one's friends. A former male client, who is a recovering alcoholic, stated flatly, "If I can't drink with Kevin, there's not much else to do. That's what we do together—drink. What else could we do?" Another complained his friends stopped calling him when he stopped drinking.

This connection poses a real dilemma for men whose occupations encourage alcohol consumption. One client was concerned that abstaining would have a detrimental effect on his business success. "If I don't drink with my customers, they'll think I'm a nerd. They won't enjoy golfing or going to dinner with me. My not drinking will make them uncomfortable, and they'll end up buying supplies from someone else."

Furthermore, men often regard addictive patterns not as problems, but rather as solutions—for stress, sleeping problems, or depression.

It is common to hear, "Of course I drink a lot. If I didn't I couldn't sleep, and then what good would I be?"; "We live in a stressful vicious world—my job is a bitch. Marijuana has a calming effect on me, and without it I'd really be a bear"; or "What harm can gambling do? My life is boring. I make a little money, and the thrill is all I have to look forward to."

Addictive behavior is due in part to the male need to feel omnipotent, which can be temporarily satisfied by alcohol, drugs, excessive gambling, or excessive sex. Of course, the sense of autonomy is illusory. As Bepko (1989) observed:

> The primary characteristic of an addictive process is that the attempt to have power or control of oneself through the use of some external agent ultimately renders a person powerless and dependent. (p. 407)

The most vital element of the assessment process is the therapist having the courage to ask about addictions. We have found many therapists are reluctant to ask men about addictions because they fear the inquiry will alienate or anger their male clients, and put them on the defensive. Consequently, their questions are not direct, or, worse, they do not broach the subject until the repercussions of the addiction make it unavoidable. This may not happen until the male client is charged with drunken driving or spouse abuse. We have found it in the male client's best interest to ask directly and early in therapy. Even if the male client responds with denial or deceit, he knows addictions are an important concern of the therapist.

Treatment Considerations

The first step of addiction treatment may well be the most important: getting male clients to admit they have a problem with a particular substance or activity, which frequently entails surmounting the family's denial of the problem. It is rare for a male client to enter therapy for the purpose of treating an addiction. He almost always seeks help for another problem, such as marital discord, job dissatisfaction, or deteriorating health, and may not be terribly inspired to discuss even these problems in the first place. Therefore, when the therapist suggests that his problem could be related to an addiction, the client's reaction is understandably resistive. In fact, he may feel that his only solace is the addictive substance: "Give up drinking? Are you kidding? The only way I can get through work is thinking about how good that beer will taste at the end of the day."

In addition to establishing limits with the male addict, it is necessary to explore the issues of control and power. The first stage of all twelve-step programs is to publicly state, "We had admitted we were powerless over the addiction and our lives had become unmanageable." This confession challenges the male creed, which stipulates that men must be in control, powerful, and completely responsible for their own lives. For many men, such an admission of powerlessness is tantamount to renouncing one's manhood. Our case loads are filled with men who are high achievers—men who hold positions of responsibility that demand control and power—yet who are simultaneously powerless over an addiction:

• Dan built a multimillion-dollar company from scratch. A true workaholic, during its growth he was in the office by 3 A.M. and worked until 10 P.M., 7 days a week. A recovering alcoholic, he channelled his addictive energy into his work, and suffered a major heart attack at 48.

• Tom is a well-respected college professor who chairs a department at a major university. He does everything with energy, enthusiasm, and a commitment to excellence. To salve his mind, he has regularly used marijuana for the past 20 years.

• Sam is a successful CPA and is accomplished at racquetball and karate. He assured me he is a wine connoisseur, not an alcoholic. It tastes wonderful and helps him relax after a busy day.

• Bill is a hard-working factory worker who likes to gamble. It was not until his wife left him that he was even willing to consider his gambling as an addiction.

To even suggest to these men they may be powerless over anything in their lives is almost blasphemous. They believe that if they are determined they can change anything. Their model is a man like Hercules hurling a spear, for whom gravity was only a force to overcome. Because they are reluctant to relinquish any of their power, it is very beneficial for them to hear other men admit their addictive problems. This feature makes such self-help groups as Alcoholics Anonymous successful; it breaks down their isolation and forces them to realize they cannot control everything in their lives.

For extremely ambitious and powerful men the addiction performs an important function by allowing them to relax their grip on their lives. They can give control of their lives to the substance for a needed respite. If they abstain from the substance they must find healthier means of release.

Men's groups can help in confronting addictions. (These groups will be discussed in greater depth in Chapter 13.) An obvious benefit is providing men a forum in which they can safely share the fact that they all lose control at some time.

This section has concentrated on the preabstinence phase of addiction treatment. Acknowledging the addiction and advancing toward ceasing the habit is an essential task, but only the first of several. Drastic decreases in substance consumption can temporarily imbalance the body, and relapse is not uncommon. Family treatment is essential to continue the recovery. The original source of the problem must be addressed if the family is to break from the familiar addictive patterns that supported the addiction.

Furthermore, for many of these men the addiction represents an intergenerational family pattern. A disproportionate number of our addictive clients are adult children of alcoholics. For this reason, it is often beneficial to begin discussing addiction with male clients by first exploring how their original family handled alcohol and other objects of addiction. If the client is willing to share his experiences growing up in an addictive family, he is much more likely to be able to consider his own addictive tendencies. Surmounting denial of the addictiveness of his original family enables him to more easily confront the denial of his own addiction.

SUMMARY

In this chapter we examined three of the essential components of the therapeutic process for men. First, we considered the complex topic of men and emotions, particularly anger, grief, and the impact of the loss of traditional roles. Second, we looked at the relationships among money, work, and masculinity, and have suggested how to help men alter work-related problems. Third, we underscored the importance of addressing addictions in clinical work with men, and included specific techniques for overcoming men's resistance to the topic. The next chapter shifts the focus from the internal world of men to an exploration of their role as husbands.

REFERENCES

Bateson, G. (1972). *Steps to an ecology of mind.* New York: Ballantine Books.

Bepko, C., & Krestan, J. A. (1985). *The responsibility trap.* New York: Macmillan.

Bepko, C. (1989). Disorders of power: Women and addiction in the family. In McGoldrick, M., Anderson, C., & Walsh, F. (Eds.), *Women in families: A framework for family therapy.* New York: W. W. Norton.

Brown, S. (1985). *Treating the alcoholic.* New York: Wiley.

Carnes, P. (1983). *The sexual addiction.* Minneapolis: CompCare Publications.

Custer, R., & Milt, H. (1985). *When luck runs out.* New York: Warner Books.

Johnson, W. O. (1988, August 8). Sports and suds. *Sports Illustrated,* pp. 69–82.

Martin, G. (1988, June). How much money is enough? *Esquire,* p. 175.

Miller, M. (1988, July–August). Tough guys, wounded hearts. *Changes,* p. 54.

Utne Reader (1988, November–December). No. 30.

Wilson-Schaeff, A., & Fassel, D. (1988, January–February). Hooked on work. *New Age Journal,* p. 42.

·8·

Helping Men
in Couple Relationships

BARRY GORDON and JO ANN ALLEN

There is a scene in the 1974 film *The Lords of Flatbush* which encapsulates with extraordinary power and simplicity important truths about male–female interactions in our society. In this scene, Stanley, a hulk of a young man played by Sylvester Stallone, is dragged into a jewelry store by his fiancee Franny and her maid of honor. Stanley is shown an outrageously expensive ring which Franny has set her heart on and her best friend is determined to help her get. Stanley clumsily tries to wiggle his way out of a financial obligation that is clearly beyond his means. Franny is alternately portrayed as a big-eyed, pleading little girl and a shrew determined to skewer her cheapskate fiance with guilt. Stanley collapses under duress and signs for the ring. In a moment that captures the true nature of macho, with its glossy image of power masking helplessness, confusion, and plain fear, Stanley threatens the jeweler to never show Franny another $1,600 ring, then struts off with the two women under his arm triumphantly crowing, "Aren't I the greatest!"

This scene highlights how the three elements identified at the conclusion of Chapter 3—expectations, underlying conflicts, and the need for differentiation—can have an insidious effect on relationships. Stanley is entrapped in a problematic situation because of common expectations about men. Franny obviously feels he should provide for her, and gauges his capacity to do so by the ring he gets her. The ring becomes a test of his love for her and his willingness to show it. Stanley, in turn, no doubt assumes that an exchange of currency exists whereby his act of chivalry will be reciprocated with acts of love from Franny, including loyalty, nurturing, cooking, and cleaning. Neither states these expectations directly; rather, they are assumed unilaterally to be appropriate behavior when a man and woman are in love.

We can anticipate that Franny and Stanley's unstated expectations will initiate a pattern of underlying conflict that will accrue throughout their relationship. Franny's push to get the ring and Stanley's foolhardy acquiescence are Faustian acts that lock them deeper into spirals of expectations and emotional indebtedness. Stanley will increasingly feel put upon by Franny's unrealistic demands, which he must fulfill in order to prove his love. He is unable to say he cannot do what she asks, nor admit that he is scared silly about how he will pay for her wish. He also is unable to assert that he really wants a sports car for himself. Instead, he reinforces her fantasy that he can do it all, and by maintaining this image he joins with Franny to create an ongoing tension over unmet wishes, unstated needs, and unfulfilled love dreams.

If Franny and Stanley could express their differences freely and accept them, they would discover they do not always want the same things. Stanley would rather buy a souped-up car and Franny wants jewelry, but they need not love each other less for having different dreams. By respecting each other as individuals they could avoid measuring their love and testing their relationship based on sameness of interests. They could instead concentrate on meeting as many of their mutual needs as possible. If Stanley does not voice his needs and Franny does not provide an opportunity for him to do so, they cannot see themselves as distinct people with individual needs.

In many male–female relationships each partner carries expectations (often not understood by either party) that have traditional gender-based origins that silently create pressures and emotional undercurrents. When such expectations are not made clear, they lead to conflicts that are difficult to resolve because they are not understood by either party. Men and women are less able to be distinct individuals, i.e., to be differentiated in a relationship, when expectations are unstated or inappropriate. Couples who cannot be themselves in the context of their relationships are unhappy and will act in some costly fashion to deal with their unhappiness. Unfortunately, our unexamined social conditioning about our gender relationships has contributed heavily to making this a pervasive set of dynamics.

DISMANTLING THE MYTHS

Relations between the genders are difficult as two people try to appreciate and balance their differences. There are many assumptions, beliefs, and myths about the genders that influence how we regard ourselves and others, and decrease our ability to see relationships accurately. Some of these myths have emerged with the growing polarization between men and women of the past two decades. Five of the more prevalent and destructive of these myths are listed below, and then discussed in terms of their impact on male–female relationships.

Myth 1: Women are good at expressing feelings.

Myth 2: Women know better how to live life, because they are more in touch with their feelings.

Myth 3: Men and women are so different they are unable to understand each other.

Myth 4: Spouses are insensitive or unloving, because they do not anticipate their partners' needs.

Myth 5: Relating between the genders would be fine, if women simply received sensitivity and emotional expression from men.

Myth 1: *Women are good at expressing feelings.*

What appears closer to the truth is that women can express a wider range of emotions more openly than most men. Therapists who work with both men and women in group situations will attest that women generally are more open and trusting initially than men, but they, too, avoid difficult feelings.

The readiness to discuss personal matters, along with expressions of caring and friendly warmth, give women the semblance of openness. This initial openness may feel welcoming, but is not necessarily a prelude to the expression of significant emotional concerns. For example, women often can be emotional *about* deep hurts, without revealing much about the source of the pain.

One emotion that many women have difficulty acknowledging directly is anger. Depression in women is commonly recognized as masking unexpressed anger. Women may unknowingly build a reservoir of anger because they are unable to express their needs any better than men. Although men tend to deny they have needs at all, women may only express their needs indirectly.

Husbands in therapy typically acknowledge that they are not good at expressing their feelings, and admit their wives are better at doing so. However, they are often put off by their wives' emotionality and indicate that they do not want to be emotional the way their wives are. Emotionality, however, does not necessarily equate with openness or intimacy. Expressing a lot of emotion does not mean that a partner is more accessible on a feeling level. In fact, sometimes the reverse is true—emotionality can push people away at times and hide what is truly troublesome.

If husbands believe they are not as good at expressing feelings as their wives, they will be less likely to state their feelings lest they be seen as doing so inadequately. If women see themselves as the primary ones expressive of feelings in a relationship, they may not be challenged to examine their own protective behaviors. One of the turning points with couples in therapy can be when each partner realizes that the wife has not been expressing some important feelings and that the husband is willing to do so. At such a point, the partners can become more accessible and open to each other.

One couple in therapy represented a reversal of the common pattern in marriages, which is that men express anger and women suppress it. The husband had been scarred by the effects of his angry outbursts in the past and, thus, avoided his own and others' expressions of anger. Feelings, in general, were experienced as unsafe territory for him. His wife, however, was overflowing with anger. Much of her anger was directed at how emotionally inaccessible he was. The therapist pointed out that her anger was virtually the only feeling she did express. The effect was that her other emotions were eclipsed and her husband felt driven away from her. This feedback challenged the illusion that she was the only feeling person in the relationship. This realization gave the husband the sense that his feelings could be valid, too. When their relationship was freed from the exclusive focus on anger—avoiding and expressing it—this couple became more able to explore their other feelings on equal footing.

Myth 2: *Women know better how to live life, because they are more in touch with their feelings.*

Kolbenschlagg's comment quoted in Chapter 3 that "men haven't learned the art of living" is reflective of the attitude that men's difficulty in expressing emotion and maintaining the relational side of their lives means they don't know how to live. First, it should be noted that in many situations women look to men to remain rational, functional, and unemotional. This, in turn, allows a woman to be upset, perhaps fall apart a bit, and have someone to lean on. Gilchrist (1987), who bemuses that she is often regarded as a feminist author, writes in her published journal:

> I like to see a man square his shoulders and prepare to take a stand . . . I don't want to be a man. I don't want to have broad shoulders or big arms or be the one to get out and fight the big cats or the invading Huns or whatever threatens us next. (p. 155)

When women relegate this role of stoic bravery to men, it can deny men the liberty of letting down their emotional guard.

It should not, however, be accepted as a perfect polarity that women know how to balance the functional and emotional dimensions of life and men do not. For example, feeling responses, which are more characteristically feminine, are not a priori the most helpful. There are many instances when immediate, intense reactions or intuitive responses worsen a situation. They can, for example, undermine another person's ability to resolve a problem or even express their own emotions. Men and women can, in fact, help each other far more by seeking to balance each other and themselves than by judging one's manner of response superior to the other's.

Myth 3: *Men and women are so different that they are unable to understand each other.*

Most couples who enter therapy have already recognized their difficulty in understanding each other. Many wonder whether they are too different to overcome this hurdle. Fortunately, in therapy even those couples that initially appear quite opposite each other soon reveal fundamentally similar ways of experiencing themselves and the world, i.e., each person needs to feel valued and respected as an individual. These basic similarities may not be evident because they are expressed in different ways, often in accordance with gender stereotypes.

The Stoddards were mired in classic masculine–feminine polarities. To her, he was too involved with his work, he was not sensitive or expressive of feelings, and he was not sufficiently engaged in family life. To him, her concerns were too narrow, she became unnecessarily upset over many things, and she was overly protective of their children.

When one of their children began having problems at school, they disagreed on how to respond. She wanted to get professional help promptly before the problem became worse; he wanted to make some extra efforts on his own before seeking help. He worried that professional help would undermine his son's independence and sense of responsibility for himself. At the outset, she accused him of indifference and being unwilling to recognize the problem. He, in turn, believed she was overreacting and was unable to let the boy handle things without hand-holding. When they were able to hear the other's underlying concerns and show they could appreciate at least some validity in each other's viewpoints, they were able to convert a seemingly irresolvable conflict into a solution that respected both views. They agreed to the husband's approach, but with a time frame the wife found acceptable. In this way, they united their mutual concern for their son's well-being in positive action.

Sometimes, differences between the genders are attributed to biological differences. A biological analysis can be used to suggest that male dominant and aggressive behavior is not simply a chosen social role, but a consequence of physiological evolution. This presents the possibility that some gender differences have a biological basis that may prove difficult to overcome.

In the essay, "Biologic Influences on Masculinity," Treadwell (1987) concluded from his extensive examination of human studies on brain-hormonal influences on male behavior that there is a physiological component to aggression that can be linked to testosterone levels. Evidence also shows that men have a broad range of biologically determined testosterone levels and that these levels can be enhanced or reduced by social environment. Thus, testosterone does not automatically encapsulate men in a narrow band of behavior.

Cognitive differences around spatial-visual processing and verbal versus mathematical ability have probably been the most widely accepted gender differences. Fausto-Sterling (1985), in a review of biological theories of gender differences, concludes that even these differences are attributable to biology-related differences only to a small degree. While it is difficult to determine how much these biological differences do affect the way men and women function Fausto-Sterling (1985) suggests that biological explanations oversimplify how development occurs and downplay the interactions between an organism and its environment. As Treadwell (1987) points out, "None of this implies that humans are captives of their physiology" (p. 284).

Treadwell (1987) views masculinity as a construct that was developed over the millennia through the interaction between male capabilities and what males as a class determined they should do. How men. view femininity is also part of this construct. Imposed on an individual boy, his masculinity will depend on a physiological, psychological, and environmental interplay. There is little support for the conclusion that a biological imperative creates irresolvable differences between men and women.

Myth 4: *Spouses are insensitive or unloving, because they do not anticipate their partners' needs.*

This belief is one of the most prevalent sources of hurt and conflict in relationships. It is often an unspoken assumption that takes the form of: "If you loved me, you would instinctively know what I need and give it to me. I wouldn't have to ask for it." As a result of this thinking, the individual does not ask; then, since marriage does not make one clairvoyant, the spouse likely misses the chance to meet the partner's expectation.

Men and women are both prone to this misguided thinking, but for different reasons. Women have been raised in our society to maintain connection to people and preserve relationships. As Surrey (1983) of the Stone Center for Developmental Services and Studies at Wellesley College has pointed out, girls are rewarded for being emotionally accessible to others. Empathy is a skill that is developed as an integral part of a girl's psychological make-up. This "relational self," the ability to relate empathically to others, which is fostered in girls, may be experienced as invasive or threatening for boys. Being attuned to others' feelings is not a skill that has been cultivated in or rewarded for most boys. Women may expect men to be sensitive with them, while it does not come easily for men to be this way. Because women find it natural to be sensitive to others' feelings and needs, they think it inconceivable that men do not relate in the same fashion. When they do not, women interpret it as insensitivity and indifference.

Although men tend to be slow in anticipating others' emotional responses, they are not devoid of concern for others. Men are typically raised with a functional rather than relational focus, but their functional side can address others' well-being. In fact, this functional mode often prompts men to have protective concerns for others and to be aware of the practical aspects of others' problems. This explains why men are often angry at women when they do not anticipate problems, such as when a woman throws out a receipt before tax time. Similarly, men react angrily when women fail to be protective when it seems obvious the men need protection, e.g., when a woman brings the man a problem when he has just returned from a long day of solving problems at work.

There are two lessons to be learned about this myth regarding the anticipation of others' needs. We like to believe when two people are in love they can finish each other's sentences and know implicitly what is in the other's heart. Unfortunately, being in a relationship does not automatically enable a person to read the other's mind. Second, men and women are sensitive in different ways. Empathy is certainly essential to satisfying relationships, and many men need to develop the capacity to be empathic, but it is not the only form sensitivity takes. For example, altruistic behavior and practical support convey caring. Neither gender is served well by unrealistic expectations of sensitivity.

Myth 5: *Relating between the genders would be fine, if women simply received sensitivity and emotional expression from men.*

It is widely stated that women want more emotional accessibility from men. However, sometimes it is easier to complain about what we do not have than adjust our behavior to help foster the desired results.

If men are to become more emotionally accessible, they need support to relinquish the traditional expectations that act as barriers. Relinquishing those expectations means that women will have to accept less from men as providers and protectors in the traditional sense. For many women this poses more difficulty than they antici- pate, as it requires attitude changes they may not have considered.

A professional, independent woman came for therapy to decide whether to marry a man with whom she had been living. One of her primary concerns was his lack of ambition. She felt guilty about having these feelings, but could not submerge her worries:

> "Can he care for me and the children when we have them? In my family men wanted to be the top; they were executives. He doesn't want to do that. He's not assertive enough, and I have to speak for him all the time."

Another woman had lived with a man for 8 years and had a good job, but was unsure about making a career change. She admitted that one reason she was now considering marriage was to be able to stay home.

When husbands do invest more at home and assume the role of involved parent expected of them, some women find it unsettling. They feel their own domestic role being diminished.

In many couples with a recovering alcoholic spouse it can be unexpectedly arduous to adjust to a sober mate. In much the same way, many women find that their male partners' responsiveness to requests for change brings its own trials. Change in one part of a system inevitably necessitates changes in the related parts, which can pose a considerable dilemma.

THE ROLE OF THERAPY

Gender-based concerns may not enter into therapy directly with certain couples; for example, couples where one or both partners' behavior is dominated by psychopathology such as major depression. However, the impact of gender-based factors provides useful back- ground and is at least secondarily relevant in the treatment itself for most couples. This section will highlight some of the problems gender issues commonly present in the context of couples' therapy, particularly with men. These gender-related therapeutic approaches can help men and women overcome the obstacles of entrenched myths and socially constructed realities about gender differences.

The impact of gender in couples work is often felt from the outset by how men enter therapy. For many men coming for counseling with their mates this is their introduction to therapy, and may also be the first situation that supports discussing feelings, needs, and expectations. Men frequently enter therapy under pressure from their spouses, often with the relationship itself at stake. This state of vulnerability can make men more accessible than they normally would be, because they are open to anything that might save their relationship. They may be more willing to try to understand themselves and reexamine values that previously were held as sacrosanct. On the other hand, the need to appear invulnerable is a strong force in men. This poses a dilemma for the therapist, who must create an environment safe enough to encourage the expression of vulnerable feelings, yet, in a sense, takes advantage of the threat to the husband's marital security that may well be keeping him in treatment.

Men who are reevaluating their marital relationship on their own initiative are usually more receptive to the process of therapy than those who come under duress. In the common situation where men are less receptive, therapy can offer the pleasant surprise of an approach that avoids blame and thus helps them feel less besieged. Men often have been admonished by their spouses before entering therapy for their closedness and inaccessibility. They expect to be accused of this by the therapist as well, since therapy is perceived to require the expression of one's feelings. Therapy helps allay this fear when it focuses on the mutuality of problems. The accepting, nonjudgmental atmosphere of therapy, thus, can often disarm the male primed to resist exposure.

When the therapeutic process can also illuminate wives' behaviors that contribute to dysfunctional male behavior, husbands receive support where they usually feel blamed and entrapped. When men can hear their problems are mutually created (as they usually are, though not always) and must be mutually resolved, they generally feel relieved. Therapy proposes a different attitude to them, which may feel new and uncomfortable, yet also freeing.

The risk of losing their wives makes some husbands more aware of their dependence on their partners as well as their resistance to change in the relationship. Facing how dependent they may be is quite threatening for most men. Though it can be a difficult challenge for the therapist to deal with this issue, the context of marital problems can be used to help a man face some of the most fundamental of his psychological barriers to change.

After the entry issues are addressed, basic skills taught in couples' therapy also require that therapists employ knowledge of gender differences. This is especially true in the development of communication, conflict resolution, and negotiation skills, and in promoting emotional and sexual intimacy within the dyad.

Simply urging men to communicate more intimately with their wives is not effective if the therapy does not recognize the difficulty men have in doing so. Most husbands know their wives want more communication, but they do not necessarily know the language their wives hope to hear. It is often as though the partners are talking different languages (see Chapter 3). Trying to discern feelings and describe them is foreign for many men. Often, men have difficulty distinguishing between thoughts and feelings. As with any unfamiliar language, it is initially cumbersome and the words don't always come out right.

Another obstacle to communication for men is their proclivity to respond to concerns with action and not feelings. As a result, husbands tend to listen and respond differently than their wives. Men tend to be functional even in their listening behavior. Husbands try to get the facts of a problem so they can help their wives find a solution. They hear their wives' communications as requests for responsibility and solutions, when, in fact, they are often intended to solicit connection, comfort, and simple listening.

One husband in therapy always reacted to his wife crying as though the crying meant he must have done something wrong. Consequently, he either withdrew because he felt guilty or became angry because he felt she was rejecting his best efforts. The idea that he did not have to be responsible for his wife's feelings and could just hear them was a liberating revelation. Learning communication, then, requires discarding old habits before new ones can develop.

Therapy can also be helpful in promoting a better environment for communication by clarifying how men perceive their own efforts at communicating. Although men are often viewed as not listening or communicating at all, this may well be due to a difference in gender language, not some form of male affective mutism. Men do listen and respond, but out of the functional, protective role they are used to and for which they have been rewarded for so long. They feel their communication has been unfairly criticized by women because they have been responding as helpfully as they know how. A wonderful example of such gender miscommunication is found in the Pulitzer Prize-winning novel *Breathing Lessons* (Tyler, 1988):

> "You don't suppose she wants me to be a pallbearer or something do you?"
> "She didn't mention it."
> "But she told you she needed our help."
> "I think she meant moral support," Maggie said.
> "Maybe pallbearing is moral support."
> "Wouldn't that be physical support?"
> "Well, maybe," Ira said. (p. 19)

Because therapy offers a nonjudgmental arena, it can support the ways men are trying to communicate, while clarifying where they need to improve.

Like communication, negotiating and resolving conflicts cannot be learned without understanding the obstacles. The belief of some women (see, for example, Miller, 1983) that men react aggressively to marital conflict to maintain their dominance over women is simplistic and bleak in its outlook. It suggests that men are unlikely to change since they will not want to give up their presumed power. This view also ignores the complexity of feelings men experience in relation to women.

Our work with men indicates they often feel more powerless than powerful; they are as frequently submissive, in the sense of suppressing their needs to please others, as they are dominant. Because men believe their masculinity requires being strong for women and because they carry an unfulfilled need for nurturing into their relationships, men are dependent on women and on their approval. Their dominant behavior is a facade. A therapeutic approach that fully takes into account the psychological underpinnings of male behavior in conflict situations has much more potential to help a man modify his handling of conflict and control situations. Men will not be open to learning different ways of handling conflict if they feel it will be at the expense of their male identity.

It is, of course, not always possible to resolve conflict sufficiently to maintain a marriage. Increasingly, though, it is women who are leaving their husbands and initiating divorce actions (Lear, 1988). Like the Frog Prince in Chapter 3, the jolt that husbands are given by their wives' rejection prompts increasing numbers of husbands to desire change—to understand what happened and what their part in the break-up really was, and to learn how to go through the divorce without acting on the aggressive, adversarial inclinations they might feel. Periods of separation and divorce can so disturb husbands that they are willing to learn new ways of facing their pain and that of their wives. In these situations, and ideally in less crisis-filled ones, therapy can teach men how to hear and respond to anger differently, and also how to voice and negotiate for their needs. For many men this is the first time they are open to such learning. For too many others the break-up of their marriage is another lost opportunity to learn.

Teaching communication and conflict resolution skills is important, but therapy plays a more substantial role in promoting change for couples when it helps them understand the sources of the behavioral patterns that govern their individual and dyadic lives. For a majority of men this represents a virginal foray into self-understanding. When men see how much of their behavior in marriage is conditioned by the past and entwined with their male self-image, they are more likely to reexamine a variety of entrenched behaviors. For example, discovering that he is looking unrealistically to his wife to fill childhood voids can help a husband understand the ways in which he acts dependently in his marriage. Such learning, in turn, promotes the kind of growth in men that supports healthier, more balanced relationships.

THE PROCESS OF THERAPY

Establishing a Gender-Based Framework

Early in couple therapy the issue of accepting differences in values and feelings is likely to arise. Examining the role that gender differences play needs to be integral to this process. As stated earlier, men and women often experience each other as speaking different languages. A key step in overcoming this barrier is to help couples see the influence of gender-based differences.

These gender differences affect many facets of male–female relationships, including communication, negotiation, conflict resolution, and intimacy. Clearly, every couple problem is not linked to gender differences. However, it will be useful for the therapist to consider the impact of such differences when working on each of the above concerns. In addition, illuminating gender-based differences can help free a couple from a blaming cycle. It has an effect similar to treating alcoholism as a disease instead of a character deficiency. Seeing their differences as at least partially a result of gender conditioning helps a couple work on their problems with less judgmental recrimination.

Presenting the influence of gender in relationships is in part a didactic task. Although this perspective seems to be one of "simply" common sense, when it is applied most couples will understand their relationship in a new way. Generally, such learning needs to take place as relevant issues arise. For example, one couple had experienced the wife's having a life-threatening illness. Renee expounded freely and tearfully about her appreciation of the emotional impact on Ronald of nearly losing her. Ronald, however, was more attuned to the responsibility he would face should she die: "I pictured myself being left with the kids all alone, and I was downright scared. I wondered whether I could handle it." Renee could easily have focused on the self-centeredness of this response and resented Ronald for not being concerned about her. The therapist pointed out, however, that women tend to be conditioned to be empathic from the time they are young, whereas men are typically raised with a focus on responsibility and action. Ronald's self-focused and pragmatic response could be seen as deriving from and yet mastering his fear of losing her. Ronald agreed with this assessment, and the support seemed to free him to be in touch with his real feelings.

It is useful to establish a general framework early in therapy for seeing the different ways in which men and women relate to themselves, to others, and to their environments. This can be done informally, but a visual representation may be helpful, particularly for men who are made more comfortable by rationality and structure. Table 8.1 summarizes some of the gender differences we have found important to illustrate to couples. Discussing how these differences impact the relationship can be a fruitful learning experience.

A more experientially based exercise that also exposes such differences is to ask each partner to carry out a gender reversal for a period of time (1 or 2 days) between sessions. Each person tries to respond to situations as they believe the other gender would and maintains a journal to keep track of these responses. This exercise requires prior discussion for each partner to know how the other learned to view their own masculinity or femininity growing up.

TABLE 8.1. Common Gender-based Differences[a]

Men	Women
Develop independence, self-reliance, autonomy	Develop and maintain relationships
Place importance on following personal dreams, destiny, and self-fulfillment	Place importance on connectedness to others
Emphasize learning the rules (what's right or fair)	Emphasize learning empathy skills and relating
In a game, it's winning that counts	In a game, it's the personal relationships that count
Emphasize competition	Emphasize cooperation
Conceal feelings (except anger)	Express feelings
See danger in intimacy; feel threatened by own needs for attachment	See danger in impersonal achievement and competitive success
Fear loss of self through intimacy; experience intimacy as invasion	Fear loss of self through intimacy; experience intimacy as engulfment
Emphasize occupational growth	Emphasize family growth
See a problem and want to fix it	See a problem and want to talk about it

[a]This table has been adapted from work at the Stone Center for Developmental Services and Studies at Wellesley College (see Miller, 1983; Surrey, 1983).

Improving Communication Skills

In the *Unbearable Lightness of Being*, Milan Kundera (1985) includes "A Short Dictionary of Misunderstood Words," which presents words that mean different things to two lovers. For example, since childhood Sabina had found cemeteries to be peaceful, nostalgic places she could go to when feeling low. Franz, on the other hand, regarded a cemetery as "an ugly dump of stones and bones" (p. 104). A challenging exercise for couples is to ask them to develop their own short version of a dictionary of misunderstood words, starting with ones that are reflective of their genders, such as "success" or "feelings," or "dependence." This can be a useful device for helping couples see how their distinct backgrounds have given different meanings to many words, thoughts, and experiences. These meanings have been shaped considerably by how people were raised in relation to their masculinity or femininity. Awareness of these differences is essential for building effective communication skills.

Focusing on the language differences between genders gives the message that dysfunctional communication is not strictly a male problem. The fact that men tend to respond in a functional, problem-solving manner, while women react empathically should be regarded as socialization differences that need balancing, not "good" or "bad" communication. When men find understanding and acceptance of their forms of expression, they are more likely to respond positively to constructive criticism. It is important, then, for the therapist to avoid reinforcing the stereotype of the hopelessly inexpressive male partner.

One way to promote a balance that neither rejects male communication patterns wholesale nor relieves men of the need to examine and change their communication is to reframe some of their statements. Such reframing would restate a declaration to reveal the caring or feeling message behind what the man is saying. It is also important when bringing out a hidden message to demonstrate the negative consequences of indirect communication.

A husband who was a physician who was quite worried about his wife's health would reflexively tell her to make a doctor's appointment whenever she complained of feeling ill. His wife received this as a cold, rejecting response. He was neglecting to tell her that he felt responsibility for her health and heard her complaints as requests to do something or at least know what was wrong. However, he felt overwhelmed by the fear that he might somehow make a serious mistake with regard to his own wife. Seen in this light, both partners could accept the therapist's reframing of the husband's seemingly unsympathetic response as reflecting caring and worry. The husband could also see how they both would have felt better had he been able to express his underlying feelings instead of focusing on what he thought was expected of him.

Reframing the husband's message required him to process his thoughts when he heard his wife complain about her health. Many men are so unaccustomed to paying attention to their internal, emotional side that they are surprised to see how much is going on and how it affects them. Probably the most difficult aspect of communication for men to learn is how to listen to their internal selves. This helps men realize what they have been actually communicating,

and what they have avoided expressing. It also heightens their awareness that others also have an internal life they may or may not
express.

An effective exercise to help couples become more aware of their
internal lives is having the therapist(s) stand near the client who is
talking out a problematic situation and speak for the internal voice of
the client. The therapist attempts to identify the true feelings behind
the client's statements. The client, then, has the opportunity to
clarify or correct the therapist's version. This exercise is particularly
effective when conducted by co-therapists, which allows each client
an affective alter ego. The dialogue can then be more fluid, with the
alter egos even talking directly to each other at times. When unstated
messages are identified for his female partner, the male is made
more aware of this deeper level in her and both partners can see that
the woman also may not be saying all that she is feeling, though she
may be very expressive. An example follows:

> WOMAN CLIENT: I was shocked and disappointed when you totally
> forgot our anniversary.
>
> THERAPIST ALTER EGO: I'm already afraid you're no longer in love with
> me, so forgetting our anniversary really played into that fear, but it
> came out as anger at you for the way it made me feel.
>
> MALE CLIENT: Your anger over my forgetting our anniversary just
> turned me off, so I went in the other room.
>
> THERAPIST ALTER EGO: I get upset at myself when I screw up, espe-
> cially with you, and I was embarrassed, but I couldn't admit it. I used
> your anger as an excuse to pull away and protect myself. I really did
> feel awful about it.

When the couple is ready they can play the alter ego role for each
other and further develop their skills at understanding each other.

It is also useful to identify the underlying patterns that operate
between the initiation and termination of common types of interaction, such as an argument or inability to discuss certain issues. As an
example, a breakdown of a common argument pattern for couples is
presented in Table 8.2.

To put such an analysis on a pad or chalkboard for the couple to see
may be effective with some men because it responds to their comfort
level with charts and organization. In any case, when men are made

TABLE 8.2. Anatomy of an Argument[a]

1. Woman tries to express an emotion or feeling
   a. Man feels threatened or criticized and, in turn, challenges the "logic" of her feeling
   or
   b. Man hears as message that he needs to be responsible and tries to "fix" problem
2. Woman tries again
3. Man withdraws into activity to avoid his rising anger or discomfort
4. Woman gets more angry
5. Man calls her names out of his anger
6. Woman feels put down; man feels rejected and unhappy with his own behavior, but not willing to admit it or be vulnerable
7. Man or woman loses temper
8. Opportunity is lost to explore and resolve

[a]Adapted from an exercise developed by R. Pasick.

more aware of their internal dynamics, they are more likely to see the value of simple, skill-oriented communication exercises and how they impact a person's reactions.

Handling Power and Conflict Issues

Many women regard men as having held power over them for centuries. From this perspective, many women conclude that a woman cannot possibly secure a fair share of power by negotiating with the very person who has been holding the power all along. A woman should expect to meet only resistance from the man and to have to meet power with power. The result is likely to be a highly charged conflict.

We believe that male socialization and development need to be taken into account when working on power and control issues with couples. Many women feel powerless in conflicts with men, and therefore believe men must feel powerful. However, because men believe they must appear heroic and infallible to women, conflict with a female partner is more likely to leave a man feeling rejected and that he has failed in some way. When men react in anger and with dominating behavior, it is to defend against this threat, rather than from a feeling of power.

The following example from a couple in therapy illustrates this pattern.

John always intimidated Carla. His arrival at home started palpitations in her heart. They fought about money more than anything else. She regarded him as wanting to be in control of all spending as a way to dominate her whole life.

When asked what happens inside him when he and Carla argue over spending, John said:

> "I become completely overwhelmed. More than anything, I work to see her happy. When she puts me in these impossible situations, I just feel like she doesn't give a damn about me or how hard I'm trying, so I get angry at her and try to take control back. I figure, Why do all this just to have her stab me in the back?"

To understand conflict within couples, we need to understand the ways in which each gender feels powerless, and identify the different types of power that are endemic to each gender. These often go hand in hand. The relationship-oriented roles of women and the task-oriented roles of men can become power bases, but these familiar roles can also pose threats to the other gender.

James was a brilliant, hard-working medical researcher. He felt inept socially and always looked to Constance to arrange their social lives. However, whenever Constance made efforts to be with others, he got angry and bullied her until she dropped the effort. Through marital therapy, James saw that his abdication of power over his social life, coupled with his intense fear of rejection by others, set Constance up to be his adversary. It took considerable time before James felt enough trust to acknowledge these dynamics and feelings. Once he did, however, he was able to convert what seemed a struggle for control into an opportunity for meaningful exchange about what made each person feel vulnerable in the relationship.

Unfortunately, many couples do not consider the underlying causes of their conflicts until it is too late. In the context of divorce, the power spheres particular to men and women can lock a couple into ugly and destructive conflict. Wives may tap their relationship-based power by turning the children against the father or controlling visitation; husbands may use their task-based power, i.e., their ability to earn money or to fix things, as leverage against the wife. It is tragically ironic that each fights for control over what each previously had taken for granted the other would handle, i.e., the children and economic security.

Just as many women do not discover until divorce that they can assert themselves, men often do not realize until they are being rejected outright (like the Frog Prince described in Chapter 3) how insecure and dependent they may have been in the relationship. Not only do men need to accept their own vulnerability and women their own power, but husbands must also accept assertive behavior from their wives, and wives must accept vulnerable behavior from their husbands. Often, men may regard anger or assertiveness from their wives as "unfeminine behavior" or as a direct challenge to their masculinity, both entrenched cultural teachings that shape our views of gender behavior. However, husbands must see that their wives' autonomy does not constitute rejection. Rather, it is frequently a turning point toward a more balanced relationship in which both partners can hear each other, even in conflict.

Henry was so upset by his wife's criticism about his handling of a problem with their daughter that he called his mother to get an objective opinion. When his mother said, "Why do you think she did that—it's because she loves you and wants you to be a good father!," it clicked that Barbara was not his enemy. He was then able to go back to her and talk out the situation. He had begun to learn in therapy that he could not always trust his reflexive feelings of hurt. Most husbands, in therapy, will verbally support their wives' psychological growth, but need help to see how they may react negatively in spite of this. It takes careful processing of events such as a wife returning to school or joining a support group to elicit the way a man can be feeling threatened or rejected by changes his wife is making.

Although many women have criticized men for not being more vulnerable, they do not automatically receive a man's vulnerability comfortably. It is not uncommon in therapy to hear a woman express a reaction such as this client did:

> "He's beginning to change and express his feelings. As a matter of fact, he sometimes tells me how helpless he's feeling. I get a knot in my stomach when he does that. I guess I'm afraid he won't be able to take care of me."

Shifting dominance and vulnerability patterns can lead to new conflicts if each partner is not kept in touch with the other's feelings as they attempt to change. Trying to be responsive to her husband's insecurity and weaknesses can make a wife fear that she is again thrust in the role of mother. When husbands ask their wives to tell them what they want or when husbands are more open and request help directly, wives may feel trapped in being responsible for the husband changing and react angrily. This is precisely the moment men have been fearing: "If I become vulnerable, how can I be certain that I won't get hurt?" The shift cannot take place without risk for both spouses and without a period of transition during which each learns to relate differently.

Some of the work on conflict, as with communication, involves didactic interventions. Men need to recognize the ways they can be intimidating, and women need to see how expressing their anger indirectly promotes conflict. This involves processing what each partner experiences from the other in anger-laden interactions. Women need to learn they can stand up to a man's anger or disagreement, and men need to learn to find a balance between overpowering and withdrawing. Instructing a couple to carry out some of their old arguments in these new ways, with coaching from the therapist, helps to change chronic, dysfunctional patterns of fighting. It can be instructive also to ask each spouse: What does power mean for each of them? Who has what kinds of power between them? How do they each use and misuse control or power? What do they each gain and lose from conflict?

An exercise that helps to raise a couple's awareness of power and conflict is to have them alternate who is in charge at home on a daily basis (see Scarf, 1987). With each partner making all the choices for an entire day, the couple gets to experience one resolution to power that does not entail fighting and conflict. Moreover, each gets to experience their own power and their partner's response to having power. Typically, women discover that they can be powerful. This can free them to exercise power more openly without hostility or fear. Both men and women often find that the man is less interested in wielding power and more concerned about his wife's reaction than either expected him to be. They also are likely to realize that when reciprocity can be counted on, power is not needed.

Shifting traditional roles within the relationship can provide invaluable learning and can break down stereotypes about the other gender. For example, having a husband assume total responsibility for certain meals or an additional aspect of child care, or having the wife pay bills or get the cars fixed, not only creates a better balance of responsibilities between them, but also fosters appreciation for the other. Moreover, such role shifts heighten awareness of feelings of incompetence and how each partner may depend on the other to fill in as a result.

It is important for women to examine how they may promote their husbands' remaining in peripheral or secondary roles. Relying on them to be the disciplinarian with the children, for example, may deprive men of the opportunity to be nurturing. To avoid the common pattern of Mrs. Inside and Mr. Outside, men must be asked to, and given the opportunity to, assume roles that relate to the emotional life of their families.

Learning to deal constructively with power and control also involves teaching men and women how to fight constructively. For too many men anger results from suppressing their own needs. This is due in part to the pressure and responsibility they feel to dutifully meet their wives' needs. A man may use his anger (not necessarily consciously) to overpower his wife because he does not know how else to get free of this obligatory feeling. Learning to express his needs and feelings generally reduces a man's anger markedly. This, in turn, relieves his wife from fearing his hostile reactions and enables her to be more responsive. If a couple can take each person's needs into account when they disagree, they can negotiate effectively and without violence or explosions. A useful exercise for couples, especially for men, is to maintain a daily journal in which they attempt to identify the unfilled needs beneath the anger they have experienced during the day.

Promoting Intimacy

As with power and control, intimacy is frequently fraught with perceptions of imbalance that lead to conflict. Women are perceived to be the masters of intimacy. This perceived imbalance can create a power struggle over intimate behavior. One client reflected this attitude directly:

> "If I let her know how I feel, I have less power in the relationship. As long as I keep my feelings hidden, she's always coming after me trying to find out what my feelings are. That keeps me in a one-up position."

The withholding of intimate communication by men should not be seen simply as a power play, however. The roots of closedness for men are found in insecurity, not a feeling of being in control. Again, we can see men trying to mask their vulnerability by maintaining a stance of being strong and independent. Many men regard intimacy as dangerous because they believe they might be taken advantage of, and thus hurt, when people know how they feel.

John was an extremely guarded individual who, nevertheless, believed he had a lot of tender feelings, especially for his family. The way he described his view of being intimate represents an attitude that is all too common:

> "I have to know someone a very long time to see that I can trust them with stuff like that. I've seen too many people use your feelings against you and try to walk all over you. I won't put myself in that position, even with my wife."

Intimacy clearly requires trust that one's partner will not exploit vulnerable behavior. Because of what men believe is at stake, many are slow to trust this way. When a behavior is not practiced, the skills to do it will wither. Men are uncomfortable with, and often inept at, intimate relating because they avoid it; then they avoid it because they are uncomfortable and inept at it.

Few couples are aware of the way their handling of intimacy can be wounding. By exploring the feelings beneath their withholding of closeness, men generally become aware that they fear their vulnerable feelings will be mishandled. They are then more likely to face this fear to determine when it is valid. It is important also to examine how wives respond to their husbands when they are being vulnerable. Often, women inadvertently react in ways that can reinforce this need for guardedness, e.g., being sharply critical at a time when the man is revealing his feelings during conflict. Simple questions that engage the couple in reflecting on and describing their behaviors around vulnerable interactions will usually provide considerable new learning. By looking at such issues together, the couple simultaneously begins to forge the desired intimate contact.

Identifying a couple's own pattern of relating around intimacy can be used to free the couple from their relational ruts. A paradigm that has frequently been written about in the literature on couples (Scarf, 1987) is that of a "pursuer" and a "distancer." Commonly, it is the woman as the pursuer who attempts to draw the man into a closer relationship. Men may resist in order to manipulate their partners, thus being the distancer, but also because such pursuit plays into their feeling of being threatened. The negative cycle that emerges is simple to describe, but difficult to overcome, particularly because couples are often blind to it: The husband remains withdrawn out of lack of trust and unwillingness to be vulnerable; the wife struggles to draw him out; the husband feels besieged and pulls further inward. One husband, Ronald, described it this way: "I was like a clam. The more Barbara expressed her emotions and tried to get me to express mine, the more I felt suffocated and threatened. So I closed up tightly."

In part, because of his male socialization, Ronald needed to feel secure in his individuality before he could be fully intimate with Barbara. Influenced by her female socialization, Barbara needed to feel connected to Ronald before she could accept their separateness. In Ronald's case a period of individual therapy proved necessary before work with the couple could be effective. Barbara's individual therapy helped her to feel she could be a separate, whole person regardless of Ronald's behavior, which in turn allowed her to give Ronald the space he needed.

There is also a dependent side to men that needs connection to feel secure. This side typically emerges when wives set their own direction out of a desire for self-growth. The relationship can become like a seesaw: the more one person's individual or "I" needs are met, the greater the other person's need for connection or "We." Understanding how their gender training impacts their needs around intimacy provides the fulcrum necessary for balance in this I/We struggle. Again, it is necessary to explore feelings underneath the man's surface reaction, usually anger, when his wife is becoming more independent. Feelings of being abandoned, lonely, or not taken care of usually emerge and can be traced to childhood experiences. Just as with adolescents, therapists may need to identify and validate such emotional reactions for men to be more comfortable in accepting them in themselves.

It is important not to see men as the only gender that is fearful of intimate contact. As Rubin (1983) points out, male avoidance of closeness can save women from facing their own difficulties with closeness. Emotional and nurturing behavior are easily mistaken for intimacy. These behaviors may foster intimacy, but they are not synonymous with it and can even work against it at times. Intimate connection in a relationship involves a high level of self-disclosure, openness, and vulnerability, which can feel threatening to both genders.

Many wives are uncomfortable with their husbands' overtures for closeness for reasons that parallel men's. If they become truly vulnerable they may be hurt or be engulfed by their partner and lose a hard-earned sense of self. Janice had prodded her husband, Alan, for years to assume responsibility for planning one-to-one time together. Because he had not done so, she never felt he was committed to the relationship. Through therapy Alan realized he held back due to his fear of failure within the relationship. When he finally accepted the responsibility to plan time together, however, Janice became tense. She said she was delighted, but also acknowledged: "It really scares me. As long as Alan stayed in his shell, I guess I didn't have to face how I would handle things. This makes me wonder how I will handle it."

To promote intimacy in couples, then, requires recognizing the fear often attached to it for both men and women. When wives acknowledge their discomfort about being intimate, it helps men to feel legitimated in their fears and helps them to risk intimacy. Therapy can create an atmosphere in which efforts at intimacy can be received differently than anticipated or experienced in the past. It takes careful processing of intimate exchanges in therapy to illuminate how the couple deals with these opportunities. When couples avoid the chance to risk intimate contact or when their responses truncate it, it can be effective to pursue how each partner would have preferred to respond under ideal conditions and then have the couple attempt to repeat the interaction in the preferred manner. Assigning homework to spend structured periods (15 to 30 minutes) of time engaging in intimate conversation not only promotes needed practice, but helps the couple overcome the inclination to avoid it and relieves either partner from having to be responsible to push for it. Some men find it more acceptable initially to try being intimate under conditions that are assigned by a professional and not self-initiated.

The turning point for men in therapy, not surprisingly, is when they find their own motivation to let down their masculine guards. Sometimes this comes with the support and acceptance afforded by the therapy environment. They discover that it actually feels good to get those pent-up, repressed feelings out in the open. For others it takes a realization about the cost of their closedness, i.e., lost opportunities with parents, siblings, or children, which the therapist may need to help them see. Often it is necessary to use the interaction with the therapist itself as a device to teach what closedness does to a relationship. To give feedback regarding a male client's interactional behavior, however, requires that a high level of trust has been established.

When men are only trying to appease their wives by making efforts to be intimate, they cannot be genuine about doing so. A recently divorced man realized all his efforts at being the kind of man he thought his wife wanted prevented his figuring out who he really was. With the most honest emotion he had expressed to her he said, "I should have taken care of myself, and paid attention to what I really needed, too. When I look at it now, I see that it was like I was addicted to you." That addiction—the hidden dependence in men on women—often prompts men to relinquish the responsibility for their own growth. Trying to maintain the man's ownership of this responsibility is a critical challenge for the therapist.

A colleague of ours recently said, "I don't think that women have license to pull out men's feelings" and went on to explain that when women do this, men tend to respond with anger out of the feeling that "women think there is only one way to do it—their way." Women must let men find their way, which requires accepting that it will be based on a masculine model, not a feminine one. Therapists, too, must operate from this perspective.

GUIDELINES FOR HELPING MEN IN COUPLE RELATIONSHIPS

1. *Recognize that men have feelings and most want to be able to express them; they are generally not insensitive or intentionally withholding.* Even when men enter therapy with resentment or discomfort, it is important to be supportive of their feelings and not simply focus on their "resistance." Reframing the men's communication to reveal latent emotion can help foster more direct expression of feelings.

2. *Do not assume men are in touch with their feelings enough to express them.* They may need help with awareness of their internal lives and the language skill to talk about feelings. By the same token, do not assume the woman is able to express feelings simply because she is concerned that the man does not.

3. *Recognize the differing intimacy needs for each person in the relationship and avoid judgments regarding these differences.* Time together, separateness, nurturing, and being nurtured are important needs that tend to be lumped together, when they are actually overlapping, but distinct. Seeing them separately can help each person understand the other better and reduce conflict over these different intimacy needs.

4. *Address the ways gender-related behaviors affect each partner;* for example, how a man's need to appear autonomous or a woman's needs for connection impact upon their partner.

5. *Identify conflicting expectations in a relationship that lock each partner into impossible roles;* for example, a wife who is working, yet expected to carry an unreasonable share of the domestic responsibilities, or a husband trying to be close to his children, yet always having to be the disciplinarian.

6. *Teach how to replace manipulative, dysfunctional uses of power with positive ways to get one's needs met.* This focus avoids either partner feeling powerless as they try to change their way of relating. As men eliminate intimidating behaviors and women assert themselves and express their anger, a reversal can occur that prompts men to acquiesce or withdraw, and women to be strident. Each gender must learn to use the options that exist between passivity and aggression.

7. *Promote equality and mutuality in relationships rather than try to redistribute power.* When men are seen as feeling powerful, women regard them as having little incentive to change. Men often feel powerless; moreover, they can be helped to give up their learned dominant behaviors if they know they will retain the respect and love of their partners in the process.

REFERENCES

Fausto-Sterling, A. (1985). *Myths of gender: Biological theories about women and men.* New York: Basic Books.

Gilchrist, E. (1987). *Falling through space.* Boston: Little, Brown.

Kundera, M. (1985). *The unbearable lightness of being.* New York: Harper & Row.

Lear, M. W. (1988, March 6). The new marital therapy. *New York Times Magazine.*

Miller, J. B. (1983). *The construction of anger in women and men.* Stone Center for Developmental Services and Studies. Work in Progress Publication Series.

Scarf, M. (1987). *Intimate partners.* New York: Random House.

Surrey, J. L. (1983, November). *Self-in-relation: A theory of women's development.* Paper presented at Stone Center for Developmental Services and Studies, Wellesley, MA.

Treadwell, P. (1987). Biologic influences on masculinity. In H. Brod (Ed.), *The making of masculinities* (pp. 259–285). Boston: Allen & Unwin.

Tyler, A. (1988). *Breathing lessons.* New York: Knopf.

·9·

Men and Sexuality

RICHARD L. METH

You are every woman in the world to me,
And every season I go through;
You are every woman in the world to me,
Especially when I'm making love to you.
                    DAVE MASON, 1973

DEFINING THE PROBLEM

Sex and intimacy are often used by men synonymously, as if they are
the same thing. Sex is one form of intimacy, of course. But if a man
wants to be intimate, does it necessitate sexual activity? Is sexual
intimacy the only kind of intimacy men learn about? Finally, is sexual
intimacy a means of avoiding other forms of intimate contact?

Clearly, some men can be intimate without sexual activity. There
are also men who claim they can be intimate without sex. Finally,
there are men who firmly believe that sex and intimacy are the same
thing.

Although most sexual problems for men occur within the context
of a relationship, the ideas and misconceptions they have about sex
develop long before a relationship begins. Although few men acknowledge it, their sexual identity is influenced by the myth of male
superiority. Our feminist colleagues have been telling men for years
about male abuses of power and control. Men are raised to be
aggressive and dominant in all facets of their lives, from the board-
room to the bedroom. They have had the power and, in most
instances, have been unwilling to relinquish it. Friedan's *The Feminine Mystique* (1963) and Millet's *Sexual Politics* (1970) challenged

this hierarchy and inspired the Women's Movement. Women began to question the justice of male supremacy, espcially in the bedroom.

As women were encouraged to express more openly their sexual needs and desires, men discovered, albeit with some pain and surprise, that their sexual prowess was not what they thought it was. In the past 20 years there has been an increase in reported sexual dysfunction among men. Some believe the increased incidence of premature ejaculation and impotence can be attributed in part to the pressures presented by women's new sexual attitudes and values, while others maintain that men are becoming more comfortable reporting such problems (Gould, 1982).

Men may experience profound conflict between what they learned growing up and what is expected of them as sexual partners now. Such strife frequently leads to anxiety and depression, which some men try to reduce by means that create new problems, including extramarital affairs.

GARY: *38-years-old, married, one child, lawyer in big city firm*

The answering service called me on Saturday morning with an urgent message from a past client. I called Gary back as soon as I could. Since he sounded so devastated on the phone, I told him I could see him in a couple of days when I had an opening. We had stopped seeing each other on a regular basis several months earlier, at his suggestion. Gary had first consulted me to address career conflicts. His problems at the law firm had not disappeared, but he had learned to deal with them more effectively. His marriage and his new role as father seemed to be going well—until he called. The night before his call he told his wife that he had been having an affair for almost 1 year. He never mentioned this in the earlier therapy.

When Gary came into my office he looked tired and run down. He immediately asked me what he could do to get his wife back, struggling to hold back tears, which poured out despite his efforts. As I listened to him share his pain, I realized I actually felt hurt that he could not discuss this with me earlier in therapy. I tried to remember everything I knew about his relationship with Eileen. They came in together for 10 sessions or so and those sessions seemed to have gone well. From what I could recall both reportedly felt satisfied with their sexual relationship.

When Gary was able to talk more calmly, I told him I was surprised he had not discussed this other relationship with me. Given the way men are socialized to conceal and control painful feelings, his response was predictable: "I thought I could handle it myself, and never realized how it was eating away at me . . . I don't know what to do now. (crying heavily) What do I do now? I don't want to lose Eileen."

The original Kinsey (1948) studies projected approximately 50% of men are involved in an extramarital affair. Since then, some of the estimates have been higher. But as Pittman (1989) points out, numerous misconceptions about affairs prevail in our society, especially the myth that everybody is unfaithful. Pittman found that 50% of husbands have been unfaithful, compared to approximately 30–40% of wives. However, a recent study by Pearsall (1987) found that over 70% of the men in his sample reported having sex outside of their marriage, whereas 47% of women admitted the same. There is no definitive answer to explain why such a high percentage of men turn to partners outside of their marriage. One factor may be the lack of verbal skills men bring into relationships. A man's inability to verbalize feelings of dissatisfaction is not uncommon. In general, a man feels uncomfortable discussing such feelings with his partner. This was evident in talking with Gary after his wife learned of his affair:

THERAPIST: I'm unclear as to why you couldn't tell Eileen of your unhappiness?

GARY: I'm not sure I know even now . . . How do you tell your wife she's not so great in bed anymore? I didn't want to hurt her I guess . . . that's pretty ironic because the affair with Randi hurt her even more.

THERAPIST: What needed to be different—how would you have enjoyed being with her more?

GARY: That's what's really crazy about this—I really can't put my finger on one thing (a long pause) . . . Things seemed to deteriorate after one of our big blow ups. It was building up, I could tell. She was always getting on my case about tennis, saying I played too much and cared more about being with my friends than with her, which really upset me. Same old thing with her.

THERAPIST: So, you were angry at her for saying that. Do you suppose these feelings were getting in the way of wanting to be sexually intimate?

GARY: I'm sure that's part of it—but there's something else which I realize now has been bugging me: Eileen says I'm selfish in bed, that

I'm not patient with her. You see, it takes her a while to get aroused to the point where she's ready for intercourse. I just have a hard time waiting for her. I also can't understand why it takes her so long, and I must admit, I wonder if it's me.

THERAPIST: Do you think you're responsible for her not getting aroused?

GARY: I never wanted to admit it, but it's probably the truth.

THERAPIST: Where did you get this idea that it's your responsibility to get her aroused?

GARY: Well, isn't it? I mean, I was always taught that it was the man's responsibility to satisfy the woman. If she's not getting aroused, then I'm not turning her on; it's as simple as that.

THERAPIST: Unfortunately, it's not that simple. Men are not responsible for their partner's orgasm, although this is what many have been taught . . . this is just another one of the macho myths men have bought into.

GARY: Great, and I've believed this all these years.

Gary is not alone with this misconception. Actually, I hear this from many men. This is due in part to a basic lack of sex education, and in part to the enormous emphasis men place on performance. It is remarkable that my statement to Gary was the first time someone challenged one of many myths about masculinity he had internalized from boyhood. Further discussion revealed how oblivious Gary was to the impact of learned gender behavior and how that interfered with his marital relationship. I suggested to Gary that one of their problems may be that he and Eileen learned different ways of getting close and different ways of getting their needs met. Although there are times Eileen wants closeness without any physical or sexual contact, Gary had never learned to get close with women in nonsexual ways. Like the man who equates intimacy with sex, Gary cannot understand when Eileen complains about the lack of intimacy. Gary's reaction to my suggestion further highlights how dichotomized gender differences have become:

GARY: Sure, this makes sense. But Eileen's idea about closeness is talking about feelings—something I don't do. It's beginning to sound like if I want a better relationship with Eileen, I need to relate more like a woman; that seems ridiculous. Why can't men act like men, and women act like women?

THERAPIST: That's a question I'd like to answer with another question: Why does it have to be that certain ways of behaving are either masculine or feminine? We all have basic human needs regardless of our sex. What happens is that men become lonely, isolated, and unhappy in relationships with women because of these limitations. It's sad.

GARY: I can see your point, because as men we're taught to behave in certain ways. But there are a lot of men out there who wouldn't buy your argument. I'm not really into being a macho guy—what I do just happens, like I've been programmed or something. But you're right, there are times I do get lonely.

Gary listened with an open mind and appeared willing to change. But there are men who are not as open-minded. Chuck, a 42-year-old contractor, is an example of this kind of man. Chuck's wife, Joan, a 42-year-old administrative secretary, called the therapist expressing feelings of frustration and despair about her marriage. In 20 years of marriage she had raised two children, and now, with their youngest off at college, Joan felt "empty." "It seems like we just exist together, as if we don't know each other." Although we scheduled a time for them to come in, Joan doubted her husband would show up. Because this is such a common fear, the first phone call can be a time to discuss different strategies for getting the husband in. It is important for the therapist to find out how the wife intends to talk with her husband about therapy, since some approaches are likely to scare men away. (For example, one woman told her husband that it was his fault that she was miserable so he had to see a therapist with her). But even more sensitive approaches will not guarantee men will attend therapy.

This was precisely what happened to Joan. A half-hour before their first session, Joan called to cancel because Chuck had not come home from work. Fighting back tears and sounding more desperate, Joan asked whether she should come in alone. I understood her need to have someone listen to her in this difficult time, but I was also concerned how this would impact on Chuck. Perhaps he would feel jealous or left out, or maybe he would feel relieved if his wife saw me alone. As I pondered the potential negative consequences of this for Chuck, Joan decided to try once again to get Chuck to come in with her. However, this time she had decided she would tell her husband that if he did not come in her only alternative was to ask him to move out and file for divorce. She told me she could not continue to live in such an unhappy situation. It was important, I told her, to convey divorce as a reality if he was unwilling to deal with her dissatisfaction.

Chuck joined Joan at the next scheduled session. One of the first things Chuck said was, "This is probably the last time you'll see me here." I hear this frequently from male clients so I was neither surprised nor discouraged by Chuck's opening remark. Joan began by presenting what she thought to be one of their biggest problems as a couple. She believed her husband was preoccupied with sex. She felt she could no longer be sexually intimate with Chuck until he realized that she needed to be with him to talk, and spend time together in nonsexual ways. She complained that their only intimate contact was when he wanted sex.

Chuck indicated he had heard this many times before but gave up trying to explain things to Joan. Chuck remarked, "Sex is how I get relaxed; it's my way of being close. That's when I can talk." Joan needed to be emotionally involved with Chuck before she could be sexually intimate, and he needed to be sexually intimate before he could be emotionally involved. Chuck and Joan reached an impasse familiar to many couples. This impasse resulted from Chuck's stubbornness, his male need to be in control, his obsession with sex, but mainly from his unfamiliarity of other forms of intimacy.

Chuck, like many men, did not learn about emotional intimacy. Our culture socializes men to avoid feelings. Obviously this does not mean men lack emotions; rather, they learn to express a narrow range of emotions and deny others considered unmanly. Competitive feelings are permitted, but vulnerability, pain, compassion, fear, and weakness are avoided. Boys learn to deny feelings that may leave them open to ridicule. This process of denial begins from a very young age, where men learn to conceal feelings from others and, eventually, from themselves.

Emotional intimacy, according to Olson (1975) occurs when "a person experiences a closeness of feelings" (p. 50). Olson and Schaefer (1981) developed a questionnaire designed to assess seven separate dimensions of intimacy couples experience, including the following: (1) my partner listens to me when I need someone to talk to, and (2) I can state my feelings without him/her getting defensive. I administered this questionnaire, called the Personal Assessment of Intimacy in Relationships (PAIR) to couples in my practice. It was not surprising to find women scoring higher on the emotional intimacy scale than men, nor that men were found desiring greater sexual intimacy. What were surprising were men's reactions to the findings.

Many of the men became angry and defensive. They felt persecuted for not acting in ways that they had been taught were feminine. Sex was the acceptable way a man learned to communicate feelings. Other means were considered unmanly and weak.

Most men seldom question the cultural myth that expressing certain emotions is strictly feminine. Further, men are usually unaware how accepting such stereotypes leads to increased emotional detachment, which, ironically, puts more pressure on sexual intimacy for all their emotional needs.

For many men, sex is the sole vehicle through which they connect emotionally without feeling compromised. Surprisingly, men generally do not disagree with this observation; in fact, they usually find it intriguing. It can be enormously therapeutic to discuss with men how restricting the male gender role has been, especially regarding sexuality. It never occurred to Chuck that he was taught to ignore and suppress most of his feelings. "What I learned was that a guy is supposed to know about sex, and that was it. Nothing was ever said about communicating feelings. Anyway, I've always been private about my feelings, just like my old man." He didn't see much of his father except on weekends, when Chuck and his father worked around the house and watched war movies and westerns together. I asked Chuck what he learned about manhood from his father. Chuck smiled and said, "My dad loved John Wayne—that's the kind of man he wanted to be . . . that was his hero. No doubt he wanted me to be that kind of man, too."

ROSS: *33 years old, married, no children, foreman, machine shop*

When Gina called to schedule an appointment for her and her husband she repeatedly said it would be difficult to get Ross to come in more than once. "You better not upset him or he won't come back," she warned. Their main problem, she stated, was "in the bedroom." It is an interesting introduction to a couple when the word "sex" cannot be used.

I was prepared to see a man who would be totally uncooperative and unpleasant. Yet Ross was the opposite of Gina's description. He wasted no time telling me about their sexual problems. "We might as well get everything out on the table," Ross began. He said Gina was the problem, and that he hoped he could help her to overcome her "sexual hang-ups." Of course, her version of the situation was quite different.

"I'm tired of feeling like a piece of meat," Gina asserted. She described her husband as a selfish, inconsiderate lover who thought only of his pleasure. She felt their sexual relationship was conducted solely on his terms, including sex on demand and sex that included minimal foreplay. She was considering divorce if their sexual relationship did not improve. Ross did not want that, so he agreed to come in. Ross appeared bored as Gina talked about her concerns. Finally, near the end of the session Ross turned to me and said, "I guess I better find a way to satisfy her, or she's gone."

It is not unusual to see men like Ross, Gary, and Chuck. But these men did not develop their present ideas about sex in a vacuum. The discussion that follows describes how men like Ross and Gary have learned gender-biased misconceptions about sex which distort and restrict their concept of sexuality.

LEARNING ABOUT SEX

A boy's sex education typically is built upon macho myths. Naturally, these create distorted expectations for sexual experiences—what one writer labels the "fantasy model of sex" (Zilbergeld, 1978). This model, largely influenced by erotic literature and film, becomes for many men the primary (and sometimes only) source of sex education (Zilbergeld, 1978). Zilbergeld (1978) concludes that the socialization of males "provides very little that is of value in the formation of intimate relationships" (p. 33).

Men learn to relate to women from music and film. Buddy Holly, one of the early heroes of rock and roll, wrote "Maybe baby, I want you tonight," words that suggested that women are objects to be wanted and conquered. The Beatles sounded a similar message in their song "I want you." The character of James Bond perhaps best epitomized the message to men that it is their job to get a woman in bed, if they are real men.

What is it that men learn? Much of it centers around the need to perform. Men learn that they must be ready to satisfy their partner under any conditions. In discussing this fantasy model of sex, Zilbergeld (1978) describes several myths men are exposed to: all physical contact leads to sex, sex is intercourse, good sex means one or many orgasms, and a man must take charge during sex. Men also learn that a good lover is someone who is responsible for his partner having multiple orgasms. Basically, a man learns he should be a sex machine ready to perform and should know exactly how to satisfy his partner. He learns that his partner's satisfaction will depend a great deal on the size and hardness of his erection.

Many of the early messages about sex presented to young boys abound with references to penis size, number of ejaculations, and number of "conquests." Sexual activity is one of the ways adolescent boys compare themselves with their peers. Sexual accomplishments are frequently discussed in competitive terms, with a language similar to that of sports. Barry, 43, provided a good example of this. A self-described workaholic, he had been quite successful operating his own landscaping business. Following his divorce, Barry decided to return for individual therapy because "things with women have not been right since he started dating again." One of the problems he identified was what he called "his overly aggressive approach to get a woman into bed." I asked Barry about his earliest memory of "sex education." He recalled two images. One was in the locker room after gym class, where one of his best friends was being teased about his penis size. He remembers a few guys taunting his friend and telling him that "no girl will ever want to be with you." His other memory was returning from a date and his father saying to him, "Well, did you score?" Barry knew exactly what his father meant. "After that, I felt like I had failed if a girl didn't want to go to bed with me," Barry later said. I was surprised that as salient as these images were, Barry did not immediately connect them to his current problem with sexual aggressiveness. Both images are excellent examples of how sexual misconceptions powerfully shape and distort the way men think of sexuality.

Health professionals who work with men often subscribe to the same misconceptions about male sexuality. A group of physicians were asked to examine common misconceptions about human sexuality widely held in our culture. Most agreed that men feel unmasculine if they cannot respond to females who initiate sex. They also thought that men want to initiate sexual contact and that men believe penis size is vital to female satisfaction. Overall, the physicians surveyed felt that sexually men were more oriented toward achievement and performance than women, who focused primarily on sharing and communication (Pietropinto, 1986). One of the conclusions drawn by Pietropinto (1986) was that the sexual revolution has not successfully eradicated misconceptions about sexuality, even in the medical community.

The professional community is surely not providing consistent messages to men about sexuality. Alperstein (1986) believes men are sexually oppressed, burdened, and isolated from one another due to complex societal forces, and notes that heterosexual men are particularly isolated compared to gay men, who turn to one another for support. For heterosexual men, others (Ellis, 1976; Castleman, 1989) offer direct advice. Especially in response to the Women's Movement, men have been presented many methods to satisfy women, though sometimes in ways that make them feel more responsible and burdened.

In *Sex and the Liberated Man*, Ellis (1976) attempts to help men understand and respond to the changes women have made, but at times does so by reinforcing the performance mandate. Castleman (1989) describes his *Sexual Solutions* as "a book for men who yearn for intimacy and problem-free lovemaking but feel confused by the mixed messages they receive from so many women" (p. 19). He characterizes other sexual guides as addressing "sex," whereas his is about "making love." His is a sensitive and informative book that men motivated to change should read. But it is a book that many men might quickly dismiss. As the author notes, "men who love and respect women, men who treat them as equals . . . are likely to be better lovers and develop fewer sex problems" (p. 27). Before men change their ideas about sexuality, they need to confront the way they view women.

Pearsall (1987) states rather emphatically that the number one male sexual problem is not erective failure or ejaculatory control, but rather the man's failure to really enjoy sexual interaction with a woman. Our professional experience supports Pearsall's research: men have been conditioned to focus solely on genital sex. This preoccupation, according to Pearsall (1987), has "jeopardized and compromised his [a man's] potential for true sexual happiness" (p. 123).

Men have always been valued more for what they do than who they are. Male sexuality emphasizes skill and performance, which become so central that the degree of satisfaction hinges on "doing the right things." Ironically, it is his preoccupation with performance and technique that limits the range of pleasure a man can attain with a sexual partner.

THE ROLE OF THERAPY

When we ask couples to experiment with sensate focusing exercises, a technique pioneered by Masters and Johnson, it is clear how difficult it is for most men to "just be" with their partner. These exercises emphasize nonsexual ways for partners to touch and experience physical affection. Although women generally enjoy this as an opportunity for intimacy, many men we have worked with find this an exceedingly frustrating experience. It is as though physical pleasure can only be derived from genital stimulation and orgasm.

Men can get so consumed by the performance of their penises that they deny themselves the broader pleasures possible with their sexual partner. Probably the most common complaint heard from women by clinicians who treat couples dissatisfied with their sexual relationship is that men are in a hurry to reach orgasm. A woman may experience her partner's orgasm as the moment that signals the end of their time together. One woman from Pearsall's (1987) sample expressed this most succinctly by saying "I know when he's coming, that's about the time he'll be going" (p. 122).

Given male socialization, educating men about different forms of sexual experience is no easy task. Raised to be achievement oriented, most teenage boys focus on how far they have gotten and how many girls they have scored with. They learn that a real man is ready to have sex with any woman, at any time, and in any situation. Adolescent males learn to lie about their sexual activities so they can meet the group norm. For example, few males over 16 would admit to being a virgin to their peers, although many boys of this age have not had sexual experience (Gordon & Libby, 1980).

One of the clinician's tasks is to help men discover how restrictive and limiting messages about sexuality have been for them. According to McCarthy (1987), males "view sex as a crucial, positive part of the marriage, and compartmentalize the sexual element from the total couple relationship" (p. 254). A sex therapist and researcher,

McCarthy believes men need to change their intimate thoughts and behaviors by focusing on three areas: comfort, self-disclosure, and increasing the range of emotional and sexual expression.

THE PROCESS OF THERAPY

Increasing a man's comfort with other forms of intimacy may be something quite alien to many men because of their emphasis on intercourse and orgasm. Being affectionate and sensual, verbalizing special wants or needs, and admitting discomfort are important aspects of the sexual relationship that men need to learn. When therapists discuss with a man what aspects of the sexual experience they are comfortable or uncomfortable with, the man also becomes alerted to the importance of his partner's comfort.

Men are socialized to withhold their vulnerabilities, and for many men, expressing discomfort about the sexual relationship may feel like airing their dirty laundry. Ironically, when a man shows his vulnerable side to his partner, she may feel he is more sexually appealing. In a session with Eileen and Gary, Eileen described "an unusual experience" with Gary while making love. We had been discussing how difficult it was for Gary to relax and let himself be touched by Eileen in nongenital parts of his body. Instead of just lying there feeling anxious and uncomfortable, Gary verbalized his discomfort to Eileen. Although he admitted this was not easy for him to do, it also made him appear very real and human to his wife. In therapy it was important to emphasize for Gary that such verbalizing was not only appealing to Eileen, it gave her some valuable feedback about how he was feeling at the time.

Men need to know that erections do not have to immediately result in intercourse. During foreplay men have been conditioned to regard the inevitable erection as a signal to prepare to perform and ejaculate. If a man remains fixated to this idea, the amount of sexual fulfillment will be limited. Yet it is often difficult for men to engage in the different pleasuring exercises clinicians recommend for them to expand their sexual enjoyment (see Master & Johnson, 1976). Usually, men respond with looks of surprise anad skepticism.

The pace of sexual interaction for men often imitates the pace of their work day—they always seem to be in a hurry. There are different metaphors that can help men consider slowing down the process. One man, for example, is a gourmet cook on weekends. He describes how much he savors a meal that has taken all day to prepare. "Why rush through it," he says, "it seems like such a waste to gulp down all that good food so fast." Another man I saw recently returned from a 2-week cross country trip he had taken with his family. He had made the same trip several years earlier but covered the same distance in 6 days. He could not believe how much he missed the first time because he was in such a hurry. When men are so preoccupied with their performance, the sexual experience can be likened to a 6-day round trip to California or rushing through a gourmet meal—they will reach their destination but with little idea or appreciation of what it was like along the way.

It is important for men to recognize how they have unknowingly absorbed messages about male sexuality. Because men "learn" about male sexuality from a young age, they will likely become defensive when some of their sexual behaviors are challenged. Exploring a male client's ideas about sexuality may be especially difficult for female therapists. This is why it is so important for therapists of each gender to understand how little participation and flexibility men have had in establishing the "rules" of their sexuality. Men need to appreciate the tremendous burden these rules have placed on them. We believe that several myths of male sexuality are important to address:

1. *Every sexual contact must end in orgasm for the male.* This only serves to perpetuate his focus on intercourse and his preoccupation with his erection. If orgasm is always the ultimate goal, then other pleasures available from sexual contact will be nonexistent or, at best, short-lived.

2. *A man must "be on" whenever his partner wants sex.* Men need to know that their partners want them to be lovers, not performers. Erections are not required for a man to enjoy sexual intimacy, although this is something most men are reluctant to believe.

3. *A man should know what his partner likes without her telling him.* We hear from so many women how afraid they are to tell their husbands what they want during sexual contact for fear of damaging the "male ego." Although intellectually a man may realize he cannot possibly know everything his wife needs, his unconscious expectations demand that he know how to satisfy a woman without her telling him. Not only is this a terrible burden for a man to carry, it

prevents him from understanding his partner's needs, and both from having a fulfilling sexual relationship.

4. *Sharing feelings and thoughts during sex will distract him and inhibit his partner.* Lack of communication may not present a problem for some couples, but in our experience couples who are able to have some dialogue during sex feel it promotes a more intimate connection.

5. *A man who is passive during sex will not be perceived as a real man.* Since passivity has always been viewed as a feminine trait, a man may not allow himself to just "lie there and relax." Men need to be confronted with this myth so they do not continue to deprive themselves of the pleasures available as a passive participant.

6. *Something is wrong when there is infrequent sexual contact with one's partner.* A man may feel something is wrong with him, his partner, or the relationship if their sexual contacts are not as frequent as he expects. A man has been led to believe that sex should be a constant thing, regardless of what is happening in his life. True, a decrease or lack of sexual contact may reveal a deeper problem in a relationship, but it is hardly always true. Further, if a man is not in the mood, it does not mean he is any less masculine.

With men like Gary and Ross, addressing these myths is the first step in a long process. Gary and Ross are both victims of the stereotypes men are scripted to enact throughout their lives. Gary burdened himself by needing to "perform perfectly" during any sexual contact. If his wife did not become aroused by him as he had planned, he became angry and impatient with her. Because he was not aware of how inadequate he felt for not arousing Eileen, Gary turned to another woman to restore his feelings of competency as a lover. Therapy with Gary dismantled this destructive myth, which he had believed for so long.

Ross was not as easily convinced that he contributed to their sexual problems. Raised to believe that a woman's job was to satisfy her husband, Ross initially balked at the idea that her needs were also to be considered. His past sexual experiences were brought up as evidence for Ross that he knew how to satisfy Gina. It was very difficult for him to hear that she was not pleased, but he realized eventually that not all women like the same things.

For both men, the key to therapy was to help them understand the myths they had accepted as truths about male sexuality. Therapists need to have the flexibility to teach and help clients recognize and discontinue stereotypes that adversely contribute to their relationships. A recent survey of men in nonclinical settings is further evidence that men are still reacting to the changes brought on by the Women's Movement (Astrachan, 1988). Men do not want to relinquish their traditional powerful role, but want things to change. They may not be able to have it all.

Letting go of old ideas about sex is difficult for men because it means giving up what they have practiced since boyhood. Yet, if men can be helped to see that new ways of thinking about sex offer more positive and fulfilling relationships, they may be more willing to let go the old notions that burden them and their partners.

REFERENCES

Alperstein, L. P. (1986). Men. In H. Gochros, J. Gochros, & J. Fischer (Eds.), *Helping the sexually oppressed.* Englewood Cliffs, NJ: Prentice-Hall.

Astrachan, A. (1988). *How men feel.* New York: Anchor Press/Doubleday.

Castleman, M. (1989). *Sexual solutions.* New York: Simon & Schuster.

Ellis, A. (1976). *Sex and the liberated man.* Seacaucus, NJ: Lyle Stuart.

Friedan, B. (1963). *The feminine mystique.* New York: Dell Books.

Gordon, S., & Libby, R. (Eds.). (1980). *Sexuality today and tomorrow.* Belmont, CA: Wadsworth.

Gould, R. E. (1982). Sexual functioning in relation to the changing roles of men. In K. Solomon & N. Levy (Eds.), *Men in transition: Theory and therapy.* New York: Plenum Press.

Masters, W., & Johnson, V., with Leavin, R. J. (1976). *The pleasure bond.* New York: Bantam Books.

McCarthy, B. (1977). *What you (still) don't know about male sexuality.* New York: Thomas Y. Crowell.

Millet, K. (1970). *Sexual politics.* New York: Doubleday.

Olson, D. H. (1975). *Intimacy and the aging family: Realities of aging.* College of Home Economics, University of Minnesota, Minneapolis.

Pearsall, P. (1987). *Super marital sex: Loving for life.* New York: Doubleday.

Pietropinto, A. (1986). Misconceptions about male sexuality. *Medical Aspects of Human Sexuality, 20,* 80–85.

Schaefer, M. T., & Olson, D. H. (1981). Assessing intimacy: The PAIR inventory. *Journal of Marital and Family Therapy, 7,* 47–60.

Zilbergeld, B. (1978). *Male sexuality.* Boston: Little, Brown.

·10·

Men and Mothers

JO ANN ALLEN

CHANGING MEN'S RELATIONSHIPS WITH THEIR MOTHERS

The Problem

Richard had sought a therapist on the advice of his doctor after experiencing "heart pains" and extreme fatigue. Medical tests showed nothing to be alarmed about. When Richard shared his emotional distress about the death of his father from a sudden heart attack earlier in the year, his physician suggested counseling. Richard explained to the therapist that after his father's death, his mother had said to him, "I'm thankful that I always have you to rely on." He reported a surge of anxiety, almost anger, at these words and wanted to get away from her immediately. He quickly added that he would not really desert her since he had, in actual fact, always tried to help her in the absence of his father.

Richard's father had been a truck driver, absent from home for long periods of time and seldom available to his growing son. In addition, he had been a drinker, something expected from the men in his family, and his mother had been silent and long-suffering, something expected from the women in her family. Richard revealed an early childhood memory in which he realized that his parents would not be able to take care of him and that he would need to survive on his own. He later extended this to becoming the caretaker for his mother to help out both her and his father. His mother often referred to him as "her little man." Women in his extended family told his mother how lucky she was to have him, and he remembered feeling proud of his role.

During the year prior to his father's death, Richard, who had been cut off from his father, had begun to spend more time with his father who had retired. This activity was in response to an increasing awareness of his father's age and of how much he had missed his father earlier. As he understood his father better, Richard experienced uncharacteristic feelings of anger toward his mother and sometimes even blamed her for depriving him of his father's attention. The other troubling aspect for Richard was that he had begun to view his relationship with his wife as "just like that with my mother." He saw himself as responding to her every need or whim, being "her little man" and feeling resentful that "even she won't take care of me."

It seems probable that the case above represents a fairly common experience in the lives of men. In the physical and emotional absence of husbands, mothers may turn to their sons, who become "stand-ins" for missing fathers. Sons look to their mothers—the only parent available—for validation and support. Women who embrace the mother role as their major identity marker, and "give their all" to it, measure their lives by how close and influential they are with their children. The children represent the only legitimate power open to them. Under such circumstances, mothers can become the model for all women in a man's eye, the yardstick by which he measures women in his adult relationships. Sons raised by overinvolved mothers often bring unrealistic expectations into marriage.

The early relationship with his mother can shape a man's relationships with female partners later on in his life. If the mother–son relationship is overly close, the son usually adapts in one of two ways. He can take on the role of surrogate spouse and parental child and devote his life to the care and support of his mother. Aligning in this way with his mother may distance him even more from his already distant father, but it also gives him some power and importance. Another adaptation is to find ways to avoid his mother out of fear of being engulfed by her. This can be done in passive–aggressive ways or in open, rebellious, angry, acting out ways. In any case, the stage is set for him to see women as either incompetent and needy or as demanding, controlling, and intrusive. His relationships with women will tend to be characterized by overresponsibility and protectiveness, which can also be very controlling, or by distancing through withdrawal or angry outbursts at the least sign of dependency or expression of need from a woman. Intimacy is not likely to occur in either situation since trust is not possible.

Some men experience overt rejection on the part of their mothers.

Many women react to being forced to be the lone parent by becoming angry or, more likely, depressed, and withdrawing emotional investment from their children. Children tend to blame themselves for the mother's unhappiness and get into a pattern of doing everything possible to please her in an effort to make her happy. Men reared in this type of situation become very uneasy when a woman in a close relationship seems unhappy or distracted, or simply needs a little space for her own endeavors. Many men feel this as abandonment or the threat of it. Women in such relationships often complain of feeling smothered and too "well cared for" by such men.

In the best of situations, men can often end up feeling rejected by or pushed away by their mothers in the normal course of development. Women have been taught that if their sons are to grow up normally the sons must separate from them and become independent and autonomous beings (Stiver, 1984). This often means that mothers push their boys out into the world, not letting them become dependent or express their desire for nurturing and their fears about the world. Mothers are taken to task if they appear to coddle or hold onto their sons and make them "Momma's boys." One woman confided that she could no longer buy her 6-year-old son a stuffed animal for a gift because her husband objected that he was too old and this might make him a "sissy." She bought him a puppet instead, even though he loved to play with his stuffed toys. So, in the many families where a son is denied the attention of his father, he may also be cut off from nurturing and find his need for it discounted by his mother, who is in charge of such things. Dispensing love and affection gives a woman power and makes her a powerful figure to boys in that respect. A man can feel very fragile at the threat of loss of love from a woman, and since he is not supposed to need it, feelings of anger and rage, and the need to control women can build up inside him.

Mothers do not have an easy time of it in our society. They are assigned the job of nurturing the family emotionally but apparently they are not suposed to be too good at it. The emotional complexity and conflict inherent in such an arrangement is beautifully described by Silverstein (1989). Speaking of the alliance that often forms between mothers and sons when there is a distant or domineering husband, Silverstein poses the dilemma this way: "If her son is to survive in the male world, he should not turn out to be too much like mother, nor should he be overly disturbed when their bond is disrupted. And if she flounders when he leaves her, her loss should not be taken too seriously lest he feel gulity" (p. 163).

Mothers are put into a bind as they are forced to suppress their own feelings and to help sons deny their emotional needs: The sons get angry if they do, and the fathers and society get angry if they do not. Men can often be helped to come to terms with unresolved issues about their mothers through understanding the difficult, almost impossible, tasks faced by mothers in raising sons and through a recognition of the long-denied sense of loss felt by both mothers and their adult sons.

The Role of Therapy

Since a woman is a complex human being, including being a mother, she is a combination of many traits. A son, even an adult son, tends to see her exclusively in her role as a mother and not as an individual with many facets. In that role she is perceived as someone who has either met or failed to meet his needs and expectations. A mother obviously influences how a man views women in general in his adult years and the expectations he has of women with whom he becomes involved. It is important, therefore, for a man to study and to understand the influences of his mother in his current relationships and in his feelings about himself. With some "coaching" from a therapist, a man can find ways to alter his relationship with his mother, settle old issues, and clear up misunderstandings.

As a man gains a more realistic perspective about his mother and his relationship with her over the years, he is freed from some of the disabling feelings associated with this powerful woman. When he becomes able to understand his mother in her many dimensions rather than in the single dimension of mother, he is able to project his new understanding to the women in his current life. The present is no longer the arena in which to play out conflicts, fears, and hurts from the past. In many cases, though not in all, there can also be a new and enriching connection at a person-to-person level between mother and man. Growth is possible at any age.

The initial step in helping men to change their relationships with their mothers is to get them to understand the connection between their relationships with their mothers and their current relationships with women. Many men feel threatened in acknowledging that a mother can have such lasting power over their lives. This taps into some hidden fears and taboos. In other cases, talking about their mothers, especially in a derogatory way, breaks a strong family rule for men. Mothers are to be revered for all they have done in a selfless way and are to be protected, never to be criticized. If a mother is perceived as denying her own needs and enduring an unhappy and/ or abusive marriage for his sake, how could a son possibly harbor any ill feeling toward her? If, on the other hand, a man perceives his mother as cold, withdrawn, and rejecting, why face the pain and the anger now? "She won't change. I'll just get angry again. I can never forgive her."

In the face of so many reasons not to and so many fears, the therapist must stress the eventual rewards of a man confronting his relationship with his mother: feeling better about himself, feeling freed from past burdens, and forming better relationships with those in his present life. The work is for himself, but others may reap the benefits of his change.

There are a number of questions that a therapist can rely upon to start the process of connecting the past to the present. The following represents only a sample of such questions:

1. How often do you have contact with your mother currently? Is the contact through visits, letter, or by phone?
2. Who initiates the contact usually? Why?
3. Under what circumstances are you most likely to have contact with your mother? Why?
4. How do you usually feel after talking with your mother? Is this a familiar feeling from childhood?
5. Do you sometimes have similar feelings in other situations? When and with whom?
6. As a child, with which parent did you spend more time? What was that like for you?
7. In what ways do you try to emulate your mother/your father as an adult? Why?
8. In what ways do you try to be different from your mother/your father as an adult?
9. What were the circumstances of your mother's life at the time of your birth? Had she experienced losses, marital conflict, health problems, financial problems, for example?
10. What did your mother teach you about men and being a man? What do you think her expectations of you were/are as a man?

These questions trigger a process that will yield information both to the therapist and to the man who is responding. The answers will generate awareness of the powerful influence of parent/son relationship on how a man is living his adult life. In many instances, a man may need to contact his mother to obtain information. That contact, in itself, often proves to be a beneficial first step toward the resolution of issues between a man and his mother.

The Process of Therapy

The initial phase of therapy is devoted to helping the client gather useful information. Let us return to Richard, the client mentioned earlier. As part of therapy, he agreed to talk to his mother about certain areas of her life in order to get to know her better. She was surprised but happy for his interest. She spoke of her interest in education, and her desire to go to college and study math. She knew early on, however, that this would not be possible. Her family was poor and she had been taught that her rightful role in life was to be a wife and a mother. She thought of herself as serious and compliant, and it never occurred to her to make decisions that were against her parents' teachings. She worked as a secretary but quit when she married Richard's father, to whom she was attracted because of his good looks and his ability to have fun, and because he told her that she was the "girl who could settle him down." Marriage proved to be a disappointment in many ways since she felt she had settled down even more than she had with her parents while her husband continued his fun without her. Richard, who was born at a time when his father had just accepted a long-distance trucking job, was treasured by both parents because he was the only son among four children. His mother talked of how lonely her life had been at times and how overwhelmed and frightened she sometimes became caring for Richard, his sisters, and the home all alone. She realized in later years that she had depended on Richard a great deal and now believed she had been unfair to him. He found the last statement surprising but pleasing.

The next step in therapy involved several discussions. Richard began to see his mother in a new light, guided by questions, suggestions, and interpretations from the therapist. He viewed her more as a person and even shifted his image of her from that of a weak, helpless woman who needed her "little man" to that of a woman who was competent enough to raise five children and manage a household with little help. He learned that she had taken care of family finances and had been able to do quite well. She revealed that currently she was making some good investments and enjoying her newly found independence.

The next step toward change was to help Richard alter his relationship with his mother based on his new insights. When Richard was able to understand that his mother was not as fragile as he had believed, he was free to say "No" to her when he felt she was seeking help from him in a manipulative way. He even asked her for some financial advice at one point, thus reversing their roles.

Another change occurred as Richard became aware of how his mother's alliance with him had contributed to his alienation from his father. On the basis of this understanding he was able to talk with his mother in a different way about his deceased father. Richard deliberately searched for the positive in his father and in the relationship between his parents. For the first time, his mother shared with him the things she valued in his father, and only then was Richard able to voice his appreciation of his father and have his feelings validated. He felt released from the perception that he was a wedge between his parents, a position that angered and frustrated him for much of his life.

As a final therapeutic step, the therapist helped Richard apply what he had learned about himself and his relationship with his parents to improving his relationship with his wife. By examining the parallels in the two relationships, Richard became less reactive with his wife and more comfortable in saying "No" to her when he felt her requests were unreasonable or when he did not feel up to helping her. He also became able to ask for needed support and help from her, which she welcomed, much to his surprise. As Richard learned to reveal his own expectations, needs, and limitations, a more functional balance and a basis for trust was struck between him and his wife.

Richard's case illustrates many of the issues to be dealt with in helping men change their relationship with their mothers. Certainly, however, there are many other situations. We know, for example, about the high rate of depression among women which is, at least in part, due to their being socialized against direct expression of anger. This may account for the feeling that some men have that their mothers were cold or withdrawn. A man could easily take it upon himself to try to please his unhappy mother—to try to make her happy. Usually, he ended up with the feeling that "No matter what I did, it was never enough."

One male client, who frequently experienced feeling guilty after contact with his mother, realized he had been taking responsibility for his mother's happiness for years and that he felt like a complete failure because she was still unhappy. One strategy worked out with his therapist was for him to write a letter to her in which he simply resigned from the job at which he could not succeed. This was done only after he had gained a clear understanding of how he had been inducted into the role, of course, and that his mother's depression had nothing to do with him. In any case, he wrote the letter but, as often happens, he did not mail it. It was enough for *him* to know that he had resigned.

Another situation involving men and their mothers that is becoming common occurs when there is a divorce between the parents. Men frequently blame their mothers for somehow "losing" the father and depriving them of a paternal relationship. Therapy can help a man open a conversation with his mother about the divorce and the circumstances of it so he can gain better perspective as an adult. The old grievances can then be resolved and, when they are, men find that they are better able to trust the women with whom they are having close relationships.

One male client complained that he could never forgive his mother because she had deserted his father to marry another man. That had occurred 20 years earlier, but he was still filled with anger and resentment. Therapy enabled him to recognize the sadness and feelings of loss underneath the anger. He was able to express those feelings to her in a letter. He added that he wanted to know what had happened from her perspective. This began a process of reconciliation and eventually led him to become more trusting with women currently in his life.

Often, if a man is to change his relationship with his mother, he must mourn a lost ideal and a lost childhood. Unfortunately, he cannot change the past and he may never be able to get what he feels he missed as a child. Getting on with his life is dependent on letting go of the past and making peace with it. Feeling anger and sadness about mothers and accepting the lost dreams can be facilitated by therapy which focuses on the family of origin.

In the process of therapy, John began to experience a great deal of sadness about the many moves his family had made during his childhood as his father was transferred from one location to another. John remembered feeling constantly uprooted and depressed about leaving his friends and schools behind. He blamed his mother for not being more supportive during those times, complaining that she never wanted to hear how difficult it was for him. She would simply say that his father was doing the best he could and closed the conversation. John was left to suffer in silence. Then he began to think about and to talk with her about how those moves affected her. She shared with him her own sadness about leaving familiar neighborhoods and friends. Finally, not wanting to face the pain of parting, she had decided not to make close friends. She had tried to hide her feelings from John and the rest of the family for fear of upsetting them even more. This insight about his mother and her reaction did not change John's feelings of sadness, but he could now understand that his mother did what she did out of caring and out of her own pain.

GUIDELINES FOR WORK WITH MEN
AND RELATIONSHIPS WITH THEIR MOTHERS

1. Most men do not come to therapy with an understanding of the impact of their relationships with their mothers upon current feelings and attitudes. An intergenerational model can help educate them about how their identities are tied to powerful mother–son experiences.

2. It is extremely difficult for men to face the anger and helplessness they feel with regard to their mothers. Doing so may violate strong family rules about protecting her.

3. It is important for a man to gain an understanding of his mother as a woman with her own life history, needs, expectations, and disappointments. This can open the way to an appreciation of her strengths as well as her struggles, which can enrich his perception of all women.

4. It is often helpful for a man to learn how his mother may have had to temper her urge to nurture. She had also to respond to the pressures and expectations to push him toward independence and "masculinity." This perspective, combined with some information about the emotional needs of children, may help him to mourn the

unmet wishes and needs of childhood and could enhance his "fathering" of his own sons.

5. Men should be encouraged to examine their relationships with significant women in their present lives in the light of what they learn about their relationships with their mothers. Settling unfinished business with mothers can lead directly to improved relationships with other women.

REFERENCES

Silverstein, O. (1989). Mothers and sons. In M. Walters, B. Carter, P. Papp, & O. Silverstein (Eds.), *The invisible web: Gender patterns in family relationships.* New York: Guilford.

Stiver, I. (1984). The meanings of dependency in female–male relationships. Work in progress. Stone Center for Developmental Services & Studies, Wellesley College.

·11·

Men and Their Fathers

BARRY GORDON

THE PROBLEM

John had come to therapy the way many men tend to. He and his wife of 12 years were having marital problems. He was frustrated and saw little hope of resolution. His wife started seeing a therapist individually and urged him to do the same after their efforts at marital therapy seemed to hit a dead end.

More than any other factor that caused John emotional pain was the irreversible regret over having made a decision to be loyal and responsible to his father by taking over the family business, instead of pursuing his true desire, a career in government. John's life was subsequently filled with other, lesser choices made out of obligation and with disregard for his own needs. He could not himself understand how he had fallen into this pattern.

During one session John was reminiscing about how his father never came to a single event during his high school athletic career. Seemingly out of nowhere, an overwhelming rush of feeling overcame John and he began to sob. The deep sense of a lost relationship and the hurt and disappointment of never having received basic support and attention from his father was actually a revelation. He had managed to bury these feelings so completely he did not realize they existed. He knew he had always attempted to be a good son and tried to respond to what he thought his father wanted from him, but he never understood that maybe he was acting out of a need to somehow prove himself and win over the father he could never get to respond to him.

John's relationship with his father is all too common a story for father–son relationships among the adult men we see in therapy.

Osherson (1986) carefully elucidates what a major barrier to male development this problem is. Within this familiar father–son pattern, however, are elements that help us to understand men and how to help them overcome some of their own dysfunctional behavior. Three of these significant elements are the following: (1) adult men often did not receive much fathering as they grew up; (2) the relative absence in their lives of their fathers led to distorted perceptions about their fathers and about their part in their fathers' unavailability; and (3) the impact of fathers, especially absent or distant ones, is enormously significant for men and can dominate how they carry themselves in their adult male roles. Indeed, the common emotional struggles men bring into therapy—high degrees of stress or anxiety, depression, low self-esteem, various forms of dependency or addiction, and marital dysfunction—can be linked in significant ways to this impact.

In focusing on the negative aspects of the fathering received by adult males, it should be recognized that this does not automatically equate with sons' negative attitudes toward their fathers. In past generations, although it was not normative, there were unquestionably a substantial number of fathers who were heavily involved, but even with lesser involved fathers, many sons cherished the time and involvement they did get and found it very meaningful. Moreover, many sons viewed their fathers as caught up in the demands of life and carrying out their family duty and love by working hard. Sons sympathized with their fathers' being away from home or too exhausted to interact. Still, their sense of disappointment was profound.

Fathers are often described as having shown their love and caring in symbolic ways, instead of directly. Work can be seen in this light. Fathers often may be excused for not showing feelings directly because it was not perceived to be in their nature; indirect statements of affection were taken as partial substitutes. One man who came to therapy, in part to examine his relationship with his father, recalled how his father never told him in words that he loved him. However, each time he drove off to college after a visit home, his father was the only family member who stood on the front steps of the house and watched his son's car until it was out of sight.

In a personal reminiscence of his father, Safransky (1988) eloquently described his bond with a father for whom he realized he'd been performing all his life:

Not all my memories of him are painful. There was tenderness between us, and humor, and a kind of camaraderie I've never known with
anyone else. He was my father: I drank up who he was like a parched
root drinks the rain—his love, his misery, his ambitions, his failures.
For better and worse, he shaped me, and gambled on me to redeem
him. (p. 43)

The unfortunate fact is that these indirect and understated messages
were teasers. They gave a taste of what could be and left the sons
(and daughters) with a not always conscious yearning for more and
confusion about why it wasn't forthcoming.

THE ROLE OF THERAPY

It is difficult enough to appraise the impact on ourselves of tangible,
traumatic events; the impact of something never directly experienced
is often dismissed outright as "just something we lived with." The
lack of involvement of a father is one of those phenomena that are
frequently minimized as having little or no impact. It is shockingly
common to hear a client discuss the death, desertion, or divorce of a
father as an event that barely disrupted the family routine. One of the
most critical functions therapy can serve is to help clients reevaluate
the effects of their fathers' role and relating in the family.

One obvious, fundamental consequence of the peripheral role
many fathers played in their families' lives was the lack of male role
models and support for the normal development of their children.
For a male, this often meant that the person a son wanted to be like
was not there to model manhood for him. Many adult women today
regret that their mothers were role models for submissive, domestic
behaviors. Many men regret that they had to figure out how to be
men, husbands, and fathers, without direct support and interaction,
because their fathers returned home from working long hours only to
recede into the couch beneath an upraised newspaper.

Adult men today, then, have their own negative learning to overcome, but they typically have not seen their relationships to their
fathers in this light. Therapy raises a different, challenging view of
what a man has learned from his father, a view that is frequently met
with initial resistance. It is often difficult for men to acknowledge
they have negative feelings—angry and sad feelings—about their

fathers. It is also difficult for them to accept that their fathers had a role in shaping them psychologically that was dysfunctional in some significant ways. Therapy may, for example, introduce the notion that they grew up lacking a foundation for the kind of confidence and esteem that is associated with their fathers' manly behavior.

The consequence of father absence in the family goes beyond the issue of role models per se. Many sons have carried idealized images of their fathers into their own adulthood, believing that their fathers were capable to a degree far beyond what is realistic. By comparison, they feel inadequate. An absent or distant father readily plays into such larger-than-life perceptions. This could occur partly because most of what the father did was talked about, not seen, and hence carried an air of mystery or magic.

The comparative novelty of father's actions at home also contributed to their disproportionate value. Mothers, to reinforce father's role with his children, might well build up anything the father did to bring about a glowing appreciation for him by his children. Fathers were not above similar behavior in their own behalf, perhaps to compete with their wives' greater presence in their children's lives. Having a deflated view of one's own ability in comparison to a father who seemed all-knowing and totally competent plagues many adult men and fuels their drive to achieve. The result for many men is a mask of bravado that disguises their underlying self-doubt. These feelings carry over to how men react to sharing in domestic functions. Husbands may well look to their wives to teach them how to carry out those roles because they have lacked helpful modelling, yet never acknowledge that they feel incompetent. When men seem inept and dependent on women to help them be more involved in domestic and family life, it is not simply out of disdain or unwillingness, but out of genuine ignorance and a lack of confidence.

There is yet another dimension of father absence that men would not likely be in touch with on their own: The egocentrism of a child leads many children, especially sons, to believe that they are the reason their fathers have been home so little or seem removed from the family. Sons will gravitate to this kind of self-blame because of the social expectation that a father would normally want to be involved with his son. The message to a daughter may be that she is not good enough or not as good as a son, if she sees her brother gaining more of dad's time. Boys experience a feeling of rejection if they have little time with their father, even if their share of his time is greater than that of a sister's. There can be a triple impact, then, that strikes at the esteem of a boy with an underinvolved father: he lacks a positive male role model; gets an unrealistic picture of his father's ability, which diminishes his self-esteem; and feels to blame for his father not being there for him. The perspective on how a man might have experienced his father as a child is another way therapy supports self-understanding and acceptance for the adult man.

Therapy can also help a man see that a father who appears to have been on the fringes of his life is really not at all a peripheral figure, but rather has impacted and influenced him sometimes all the more by his very distance. Men measure themselves to a considerable degree, unconsciously, not only by what they saw in their fathers, but also by what they thought their fathers saw in them. A silent or distant father may well have unintentionally conveyed the message to his son that he did not care that much or that other things were more important. To a young son this would likely have been taken as a statement that he was not good enough to merit more attention. On the other hand, when a father had little involvement in the family but was frequently critical when he was interacting with his children, the power of that criticism was magnified. This is unfortunately a common pattern among fathers who return from long work days with low tolerance for the demands of home life.

In a workshop for therapists called "Men: The Challenge of Change," conducted by some of the authors of this book, the participants were asked near the end to relate stories about their fathers. One by one participants reminisced, and although some of the memories were of warmth and shared intimate moments, most were of the sense of missed opportunities and a painful loss. Most of the group had fathers who were unable to be truly intimate, yet were clearly powerful influences within their families. The free-flowing of tears and the mounting, almost tangible feel of heartache told a critical story: as adults these people continued to love and long for the fathers by whom they felt emotionally and even physically abandoned.

Therapy with men must go beyond examining the impact of fathers to helping men face and deal with the sense of loss they feel around their fathers. In part, this involves recognizing the need to grieve such a significant loss. It also means examining ways to overcome the distance established in the past. Helping men to free themselves from the emotional residue of the dysfunction in their relationships with their fathers—the anger, guilt, sadness, etc.—is a necessary step in this process. Often, the therapist must overcome the men's disbelief that anything could change with their fathers. Sometimes the feelings of intimidation that reverberate from childhood make any efforts in the present feel too risky for the men. Overcoming barriers between them and their fathers, even those posed by death and physical or emotional distance, is a major challenge in therapy and, not uncommonly, a turning point in the process of change for men. Perhaps more critical, however, is fostering the realization that, regardless of one's relationship with his father, the man can and needs to change how he relates to himself.

THE PROCESS OF THERAPY

Tom was one of the victims of a father who was extremely distant even though Tom literally grew up around him. Tom had started going to work with his father practically when he was old enough to walk and had worked as hard as he could to impress his father. At age 32, he told his therapist, "I've never once heard from my father that I'm a good worker and know what I'm doing. And now I'm having cold sweats in the middle of the night because I can't believe in myself." He sighed with both relief and regret and announced, "There! It only took me 30 years to come face to face with that." It had taken Tom weeks in therapy to even connect his father's way of dismissing and demeaning him with the intense anxiety attacks that he was having. It was not an irony to be overlooked that Tom's anxiety attacks started occurring the last few months before the birth of his first child, when he would take on the mantle of fatherhood, a role for which he felt wholly unprepared.

One of the early and critical steps in therapy with men is getting them to examine their relationships with their fathers and to see a connection between how their fathers related to them and how they now relate to themselves and others. Many men are initially resistant to looking at the past at all, to focusing on their fathers, or to linking their present behavior with either. Some prefer to block out or deny the pain, while others simply do not recognize that it made a difference in their lives. A common fatalistic outlook is that fathers could not be other than distant, uninvolved, or hypercritical, and thus having such a father is one of life's inherent traumas to which one must resign oneself. Sometimes this reluctance to look at their fathers comes from having heard years of criticism of their father's failures from a frustrated mother or siblings. To see the negatives in the father is then experienced as an act of disloyalty and allying against him. Men frequently deny or remain out of touch with uncomfortable feelings, and they do this with their feelings about their fathers as well.

With all the aversion attached to it, the exploration of a man's relationship with his father must not feel like a frontal assault on either the father or the quality of the relationship. Neutral questions that elicit a description of the father's character and his own history are an effective means of entry to the subject. Delineating the father's relationship with his own father provides an intergenerational perspective that sheds light on the father's behavior and makes it more difficult to view him in a simplistic, polarized fashion. An intergenerational focus also injects the sense of patterns being learned and transmitted. This defuses some of the tendency of the client to blame his father for past transgressions or to assume the therapist is doing so.

By maintaining a neutral stance during the initial history-taking, the therapist can listen for the strengths perceived in the father as well as the areas of pain and disappointment. The positive side of the relationship can then be validated, and feelings of love and respect affirmed. It is also instructive to explore what the father's own struggles would have been during the time he was responsible for raising this child. This process, in turn, frees the individual to acknowledge more openly and honestly the true character of his paternal relationship. When a man can be helped to see that he can still love his father and yet look at his flaws, he can also begin to be relieved of burdensome feelings. He can also start to see his own weaknesses in a new light.

Frank had come to therapy because of his frustration with his out-of-control anger and inability to accept the limitations imposed by a physical disability. He was so excited after a session that had brought out his father's abusive and demanding behavior toward him that he became committed to therapy at a point when he was about to say he really did not need it. Frank knew his father had a "bad temper," but out of loyalty and the fear of facing his negative feelings toward his father he had refused to acknowledge what that temper had done to him. He said to his therapist with obvious relief and appreciation, "You opened my eyes to something I never connected to who I was. It makes my own temper seem so much tamer by comparison, and yet I feel more optimistic and motivated about getting a handle on it."

Many men do not readily acknowledge that who they are as adults has much to do with how they were raised. They would like to believe they are self-made and self-sufficient. To help them make these translations the therapist may need to move from a neutral stance to a didactic one, essentially teaching the client about the emotional needs of children and the impact of parental treatment on a child's self-concept and behavior. To overcome the skepticism such psychologizing of life engenders in many men it helps to offer concrete, believable examples. Sometimes these can be found in present-day experiences of the client with his parents or with another significant person. Often it is easier for a man to see such responses in his own children or in his siblings as youngsters.

Identifying a father's role in important developmental junctures in the client's life is a further means of establishing the impact of one's father. Events such as graduations, school successes, family losses, and separations are rich emotional experiences in a child's life and thus serve to highlight what they may have learned on an emotional level from their parents. The father who stood on the steps longingly watching his son go off to college, but never told his son directly of his love for him, gave a complicated, confusing message about love, expression of feelings, dealing with separation, and silent bonds. Examining such moments in therapy not only helps a man understand how he was shaped emotionally, but also offers a baseline from which to comprehend his adult responses to parallel circumstances.

Phil had grown up on a farm with a father who seemed critical of everything he did and who was explosively angry, to the point of giving brutal beatings. Through therapy, Phil began to understand the connection between his emotional closeness, his fear of being hurt, and his fear of his own anger, which he believed would be as uncontrolled as his father's. He could see how his avoidance of intimacy and of conflict was playing out in his marital relationship the continuing effects of his abusive father. He also learned how his perfectionist pattern at work reflected a long-standing strategy he'd evolved to ward off the criticism and punishment he was used to and expected, and how that strategy served to cover an unrelenting anxiety about not being good enough no matter how hard he tried. Behind every supervisor's watchful eyes he felt the short-fused judgments of his father and the piercing pain of his strap.

It was a slow and difficult process for Phil to look at himself in respect to his relationship with his father. The effect of doing so was to alter how he looked at his own self-worth and his need to express himself and free himself emotionally, and to stop abusing himself in his work life. He worked hard at being open about his feelings and not avoiding his wife's, especially her anger. He ultimately quit his restrictive, overdemanding job to take a new position that allowed him considerable latitude to guide his own work and the opportunity for much more fun and professional reward. Not surprisingly, this new position took him back home, near where his father lived.

Probably the most critical piece of learning in Phil's exploration, the learning that seemed to allow for, or at least greatly foster, all the other growth was that he began to see his father as a person and not an overpowering, inhuman tyrant. He realized that his father had himself been abused and that his father had lived on the edge of foreclosure for a number of years. He saw also that his father had become a better father to the younger children in the family when the pressures of his life had subsided. In a session after a return trip to his home state in preparation for his move and new job, Phil talked about his desire to finally get to know his father and his desire to let go of his old anger:

> "I looked at my father, really looked at his face and his eyes, for the first time ever. As I sat across from him, I could see he was a simple, sad man, and he looked so frail to me. I couldn't imagine telling him how he'd hurt me as a kid. And part of me still lived in fear, despite how frail he looked, that I'd say something wrong and he'd get angry and try to beat me."

In that experience Phil really came to understand the power of his father in his life.

Discovering oneself in the context of one's relationship to his father is just that—discovering oneself. It means uncovering painful, uncomfortable feelings and realizations. These new awarenesses may lead to a man coming to terms with sides of himself from which he has tried to hide, often through various dysfunctional behaviors. There is also a positive side to this exploration. Men discover undeveloped sides of themselves and get in touch with strengths and valued qualities they can connect with their fathers. Typically, the understanding, acceptance, and self-growth of this process leads men to desire a renewed or altered relationship with their fathers.

One of the most powerful steps a man can take to deal with and heal from the dysfunctional aspects of his relationship with his father is through initiating one-to-one contact with his father. However, before a man is ready to work directly at altering his relationship with his father, he needs to have vented and gained perspective on the reservoir of hurt and anger he may have stored up. To accomplish this the usual discourse of therapy is effectively augmented by exercises that engage the client in recall of the past: role plays and written dialogues or letters that provide a vehicle for expressing indirectly the buried feelings carried toward the father. The safety of such indirect means helps men become more comfortable with their feelings and prepares them to approach the direct interactions that may follow in a constructive manner.

When Frank felt freed enough from his anger at past actions of his father, he was eager to test the possibilities of an adult relationship with him. As an initial step he chose a safe vehicle for time together, asking for help to remodel his basement. In the course of this "productive" time, his father slipped out with a term of endearment, calling him, "Dolly," a name he had not used since Frank was a toddler. That one word of affection initiated a transformation in their relationship, because it altered Frank's basic assumption about how his father felt about him.

Of course, establishing or reestablishing contact on an intimate basis with a father is not always possible and, when possible, not necessarily easy. Moreover, such contact is not usually magically healing, but rather begins a process that may have only limited potential. One man, whose father virtually abandoned the family after his parents got divorced, took several months to work up the courage to ask his father to golf with him. Golfing with his father had been one of the few positive memories he'd retained. The event took place with symbolic perfection on Father's Day and went without a hitch, except for the fact that it was utterly boring. They had little in common, and the man's father was just as narrow-minded in later life as he had been before. The tangible outcome was a decision to maintain occasional contact to keep the relationship alive, but the more important result was a feeling of being unburdened from the years of anger, guilt, disappointment and feeling cheated that came as baggage with the abandonment by his father. Having the opportunity to discover and express the painful feelings connected with his father was more important than changing the relationship in this case, because it was essentially all that was possible.

The entire process of examining and working on a man's relationship to his father helps him to see his father more clearly for who he was, both in terms of strengths and weaknesses; this, in turn, immeasurably aids a man in his efforts to understand and accept himself. Tom, Frank, and Phil are all examples of men who carried considerable tension and anxiety because of the unrealistic expectations they had developed from the framework of their fathers' examples and teachings, but they were all the more distorted by the code of silence by which they were conveyed and which they then required. Fathers not talking to sons about what their lives were really like, about the very real pressures and fears they carried, gave their children a false message about the emotional price of being male. These adult sons, then, grew up believing they should fulfill with complete self-assurance their fathers' model of being responsible, a good provider, strong, and able to compete with other men. Having self-doubts was unmanly and not something to talk about or acknowledge. Being helped to recognize that fathers, too, must have carried such doubts, and in fact acted in dysfunctional ways because of those doubts, gives a man permission to have such feelings himself. It lightens the load of being male and puts it in perspective.

When fathers who have engendered strong negative feelings by their abusiveness or distance are seen in the context of their human frailties, it allows their sons to be more accepting of their positive traits. Phil could see that his honesty, conscientiousness, and willingness to work hard came from his father. Frank could feel the love he had for his father once he could acknowledge the rage as well.

Often adult sons are confused by a mixed reaction from their fathers in response to their successes. For example, sons taking over family businesses from their fathers are frequently befuddled by the ambivalence they find in their fathers and interpret it as a lack of confidence in them or rejection. Again, seeing their fathers as having their own weaknesses allows men to shed the mantle of feeling inadequate because of the messages they have received. It also fosters greater empathy for their fathers, which can lead to improved relationships.

Another major dividend for a man examining his relationship with his father is that it can allow him to work at being the kind of father he wants to be, unfettered by the rules for manhood and fatherhood with which he grew up. Realizing that one's own father was struggling with these roles rather than being all-knowing and omnipotent can allow one to struggle also, and to see that father's way was only *his* way, not the only way to be a father. It also frees a man to consciously decide what he does not want to do as a father, rather than reject his father's parenting indiscriminately, out of a residue of anger and hurt. Since we generally end up parenting more like our parents than we expect to, this can, then, ease our self-rejection when we discover that the "apple doesn't fall far from the tree." Through approaching the role of being a father as a growthful experience involving self-discovery, a man can open the door to a richer experience for himself and his family. He can also potentially create new opportunities for understanding and altering his relationship with his own father.

GUIDELINES

1. The use of an intergenerational model in therapy, i.e., exploring a man's relationship with his father, as well as the role of grandfathers, is essential for achieving self-understanding and a full appreciation of how one's masculine identity has been shaped.

2. A realistic picture of his father and how he was impacted by him is necessary for a man to assure that efforts to improve the relationship are functional. Overcoming the belief about fathers being omnipotent, infallible, or even totally rejecting is one level of this effort. Attempting to understand their fathers' emotional dilemmas and concerns, despite their lack of expression, is another critical level.

3. Men need considerable help to recognize the sense of loss they feel from having had a distant, unsupportive father. There is a grieving process men must be guided through so they can reach the point of acceptance of what they have lost and what this has meant to them. Part of this grieving involves an uninflated appreciation for what their fathers did pass on to them.

4. Promoting meaningful, one-to-one contact with his father is the most direct and powerful route to clarity that a man can achieve about the impact of his relationship with his father, as well as being an effective means of overcoming the emotional barriers carried over

from a past dysfunctional relationship. Even with fathers who are deceased, it is important to creatively find ways for a man to reconnect with his father.

5. It is not always possible for a man to establish constructive contact with his father, but valuable learning takes place in coming to terms with this reality.

6. The exploration of one's relationship to his father can be used to help a man determine the kind of husband, father, friend, etc. he wants to be. Conversely, examining how a man operates in these various roles and linking it to his relationship with his father is an essential part of the self-exploration from which men grow.

REFERENCES

Osherson, S. (1986). *Finding our fathers: The unfinished business of manhood.* New York: The Free Press.
Safransky, S. (1988, May/June). Legacy. *The Family Therapy Networker*, pp. 42–43.

·12·

Being a Father

BARRY GORDON

- *A group of men at a recreation center sit in a circle singing nursery rhymes while they cuddle their bubbling toddlers. Passersby ogle through the window at the charming scene.*

- *In a crowded mall, a man plops his infant son on a bench and begins to search through a jammed bag for his diaper supply.*

- *A young lawyer nervously approaches a senior partner with a request for two weeks of paternity leave.*

THE PROBLEM

The above are scenes of American fatherhood that have become increasingly common. It warms our hearts to see these fathers involved with their children. With the powerful impact of the Women's Movement, there is a growing expectation that fathers will shoulder their share of child-care responsibilities. What we find, however, is a mixed response. In some areas of the country there has been enough attention to father involvement in child care to get changing stations installed in public men's rooms. The rise in men participating in the births of their children through presence in the delivery room has been startlingly dramatic over a relatively short period of time, from 27% in 1973 to 79% in 1983 according to one national survey (Osherson, 1986). Yet, in the same year that four-fifths of fathers were found in the delivery room at birth, half the fathers who were divorced were having no contact with their children by the time their children were early adolescents; only 20% of the children of divorce in this survey saw their fathers once a week or more (Osherson, 1986).

Do men, after all, truly want to be involved with the care and raising of their children, or are they simply drawn by the excitement of a child coming into the world? One author suggests that men are still not internalizing their parenting role. Part of why this may occur can be due to mothers filling in for the fathers' avoidance and making it easy for their husbands to rely on their wives for the care of their children (Rubin, 1983).

Additionally, society at large collaborates in undermining how men approach their role as fathers. For example, it is a common experience for the father of young children, upon being discovered home alone with his kids by a friend, to be greeted with the exclamation, "Oh, you're babysitting!" This is often said, especially when it is a friend of his wife's, as though it is one of the cutest things in life next to a baby's smile. Many men accept this picture of their role without realizing the psychological and practical impact of seeing themselves in a subordinate and substitute role.

The father who "babysits" his children tends to do what is necessary, but puts off decisions or initiating new or unfamiliar activities. He may well interact playfully with his children and be enthusiastic, but he may also in the back of his mind be waiting for the mother's return and feel somewhat like he is killing time in the interim. The man who tells the caller that he is not babysitting, but is simply being a father to his children, does not regard himself as being in a secondary role and is more inclined to be invested fully in the life of his children. Changing the language we use with regard to the functioning of fathers is one step in the direction of strengthening this role. As we have seen in Chapter 4, both men and their children benefit when fathers embrace their role. When they do not, there are likely to be serious consequences: The psychological well-being of the children is undermined; children experiencing emotional problems cannot be helped as effectively; an emotional and practical imbalance occurs which adds stress and leads to conflict within a marriage (or even after a divorce); and the emotional development of the father is truncated.

THE ROLE OF THERAPY

As cited in Chapter 4, there are men who come to therapy because of concerns about their children and their relationship to their children. Many divorced or divorcing fathers are particularly sensitive about maintaining their relationships, though we have also noted shockingly high numbers who do not follow through with regular contact. Commonly, fathers are drawn into therapy because of problems their children are having. Family therapists know that more often than not these problems attributed to the children are symptomatic of larger relationship problems in the home.

Often the initial task of therapy in working with men vis à vis their role as fathers is to overcome their resistance to seeing that they are part of the problem. This problem is not unique to men, but the functional outlook from which men so commonly operate makes it difficult for them to see their child's overt problem in a relational context. Establishing how relating in the family contributes to symptomatic problems is a critical didactic function of therapy with men.

Timmy was an extremely bright, though shy 15-year-old. His parents were both talented people who were heavily involved in their careers. Timmy had adapted over the years to his parents' unavailability by hardening himself into a sullen, self-sufficient loner. His parents reacted by leaving him alone, because that was what they thought he wanted. When Timmy began stealing small objects at school, his parents were shocked. When the therapist interpreted Timmy's behavior to them as the only way that Timmy could cry out for their attention, which he so badly needed, they were yet again dumbfounded. It was difficult for these highly functional, intelligent adults to connect Timmy's stealing with a need for their attention. Perhaps more confounding to them, especially to Timmy's father, was the idea that they could mean that much to Timmy. Even when Timmy himself could finally voice these feelings, it was hard for his father to believe the parents were really part of the problem or that Timmy really wanted more time with him. The therapy was most helpful in this case probably because it enforced some regular time together with his parents for Timmy and focused attention on the fact that he was not as self-sufficient as he tried to appear.

An important part of overcoming resistance by men to a broader focus on their children's problems is to help them see that, in fact, they do matter to their children. Men tend to believe that what they *do* for their children is what is needed by them, and they then relegate attention and nurturing to mothers to give. They do not readily see that their direct involvement with their children is far more important. For many this is a rationalization that they use to resolve the dilemma between feeling the demands of work and their provider role, and the desire or sense of obligation to be with their families. In therapy they can be encouraged to face this dilemma directly.

One way to help men understand their lack of internalization of the parent role is to guide men to see that they may be repeating in their conjugal families what they observed their own fathers do in their family of origin. Men may recreate a less than fully involved role because it is familiar and it is what they learned. Most men did not experience a fully involved father and, in essence, were not taught how to be one.

It should also be seen that many men today allow their fathering role to be secondary in their lives by default rather than choice. Osherson (1986) reports that there is some research evidence that men, too, have a difficult time with the "empty nest syndrome" when their children leave home. This is suggestive of the fact that men want to be around their children and are emotionally invested in them, even if they do not push themselves to be equally integral to their care.

Examining how a man carries out his role as father can be a relevant issue for men who are discovering that their attitudes about work are dysfunctional. Focusing on their desire to be a "good" father and on how they are needed at home provides leverage to engage them in examining their priorities and the total impact of their work behavior. For men who are discovering or struggling to overcome the blocks to intimate relating with others, committing more fully to involvement with their children can be a nonthreatening, satisfying means to growth in the area of interaction with others.

Both in family work and in individual therapy, it is essential to tap the latent desire by men to be nurturing. When attention is focused on these feelings few men disavow them. Helping men see that it does matter to them and not just their children to be involved as a father is an important growth step for men. This perspective places father involvement in the context of relational, and not just functional, significance. Often it requires pushing men to commit time and restructure their lives as a part of the therapy. Once the commitment begins to be carried out, the rewards of increased involvement generally secure behavior change and make further prodding unnecessary.

THE PROCESS OF THERAPY

Larry was a very intense man and was as intense about being a father as he was about his work, except that he gave disproportionately more to work. He often went on camping trips and biking excursions with his two sons and gladly took time off from work for school conferences or to see the boys' sporting events. However, he also worked 12-hour days routinely and came home too stressed and exhausted to deal with the almost daily school problems of his younger son, Larry, Jr.

When Larry was involved, he was all there, and he was as interested and as affectionate a father as anyone could hope to be. However, when his wife raised the point at a family therapy session that Larry's involvement was there when it was convenient for him, but not necessarily always when it was needed, he was hurt and angry. When Renee asked her husband how often he thought on his own about the child-care needs of the boys, he had to admit:

> "I never really gave it consideration, but Renee is the one who keeps track day to day of what the boys need. I probably never wake up in the morning and review to myself what will be happening to the boys and consider if everything is covered. I rely on Renee to let me know.
>
> "I suppose that isn't really fair, but then how much can I have on my mind at once? I think it says a lot that I'm willing to leave the office no matter what anyone says to be at a lot of the things I attend. Believe me, you don't win medals at the office for doing that."

Larry's father had been a hypercritical man who constantly worried about money and, as a result, worked every hour he could and was not there much for Larry. When he was there, Larry usually wished he was not because of how critical and short-tempered he was. In Larry's view of himself, he had made great strides in being a better father than his own father had been. Measured by this standard, rather than by what it takes to be a good parent, he was right.

By incorporating Larry's own father's relationship to him in the therapy, it gave perspective to both Larry and Renee. She could see that Larry was trying hard to be an involved father, but that he had some formidable barriers to overcome that were not of his own making. Larry, in turn, saw that he was misinterpreting Renee's motivation in wanting him to be more involved, because he still read into her feedback his father's relentless criticism. Moreover, because it was so important to Larry that he be a good father, focusing on where he could strengthen this role was well received once he understood his defensiveness.

Larry was encouraged in therapy to reexamine his work commitments and the ways he was dealing with stress. When Larry's own values about the kind of father he wanted to be were compared with his attitudes about work, he was able to see that his time and energy commitments were not fitting his own priorities. It became clear that his work stress was interfering with his father role. In addition to restructuring his work life, Larry came to realize, with Renee's support, that he could ask for help. By allowing himself to relinquish some of his distorted sense of having to be personally responsible for so much, he found he could have more time for Larry, Jr. without more pressure. The enjoyment he got from his contact with his son actually made his life more satisfying.

Most men, as with Larry, do not come to therapy to examine their own role as a father. Whether the issue arises as a result of a symptomatic or troubled child, or conflict with his wife over his role at home, or as a natural outgrowth of self-examination, it is all too common for husbands to be initially uncomfortable and resistant to looking at how they behave as fathers.

The example of Larry is representative of the basic steps that are effective in therapy to help overcome resistance and enlighten the exploration of a man's role as a father. Such exploration is useful in establishing the possible connection between a father's relationship to his children anad symptomatic problems displayed by the children, as well as the connection between that relationship and marital conflict. Moreover, there are often causal connections between a man's behavior as a father and his emotional state. For example, Feldman noted in Chapter 4 that a father's estrangement from his children can be a source of depression. Conversely, for a depressed or anxious man or a man with unresolved emotions about his own parental relationships, how he conducts himself as a father may well reflect and be symptomatic of his own emotional problems.

A starting point that is less likely to create defensiveness in a male client is to establish what kind of father he wants to be and feels he is before examining problems connected to his role as father. Men are so often underinvolved as parents that it is easy for therapists to operate from the assumption that a man is shirking his responsibilities to his children. Most men consider it among their highest priorities to be a good parent, but define this role in material terms which allow them to escape the internal dilemma of how to be a good provider and an involved parent simultaneously. By communicating an attitude that accepts men as wanting to be good fathers, the therapist can create a setting where the stresses of being a modern-day father can be expressed and understood, even as basic assumptions about a father's contribution are called into question.

Taking a thorough history of a man's experience with his own father illuminates how he came to define his own way of being a parent in a manner that is usually nonthreatening. Invariably such a dialogue reveals behaviors that a man shares with his father, some regrettably, and ones that he has purposefully tried to avoid or reverse. There is also an opportunity in this therapeutic step to do some educating about what kind of needs children have in relation to their parents and what happens when such needs are not met. It is common for men to accept as a given fact of life that their fathers were relatively unavailable, taught them little, or were intimidating. Since such behaviors were presumed to be normative, they were presumed to not be damaging. Males, in general, are not raised with attention to caretaking and nurturing behaviors, and this helps make them comparatively insensitive as adults to the effect of inadequate parenting. Helping them understand the developmental needs of children and how parents impact on children will shed light on their own development and foster more enlightened parenting with their children.

Thus, whether a man has come to therapy because his child is experiencing problems or because he is, learning more about parenting is emancipating. As Feldman has noted in Chapter 4, men carry considerable anxiety about their role as father. The lack of effective modelling obviously contributes heavily to this anxiety. Moreover, with new knowledge and skills, men are more comfortable playing an active role as parents. Involvement as a father helps them feel better about themselves and have a satisfying channel for expressing their nurturing side, which may well have been dormant and repressed, but is not absent.

Peter was pressed to seek therapy by his boss because of an erratic work pattern and difficulty dealing with an overbearing supervisor. A careful exploration of his family of origin revealed a father who was superficially a model parent, but in actuality judgmental, controlling, and distant. The more Peter examined his relationship with his father, the more he saw elements of his father in his supervisor and a pattern of avoidance in his own behavior similar to what he had employed with his father. Unfortunately, on the job Peter's avoidance of his supervisor had a functional side to it, i.e., he could avoid criticism, and it was, therefore, difficult to change the behavior.

It became evident that out of fear of being like his own father with his young son, Peter was avoiding that relationship as well. This realization jolted Peter because he was clear it was leading to an outcome he abhorred. By helping Peter be aware of his actions as a father and giving him a homework assignment to begin spending one-to-one time playing with his son, Peter began to make a dramatic turnaround in his ability to assert himself in interactions with others. He was painfully aware that he did not want to be a negative role model for his son any more than he wanted to be cut off from him.

When Peter initially tried to carry out his assignment to play with his son, he did not know how to begin; child play was that foreign to him. The therapist suggested he let his son teach him a game, which in fact worked well for both father and son. Many men need concrete guidance to help them in relating to their children. They may need background information to help them adapt their expectations and interactions to the child's needs. They may need ideas and practical advice on how to be with their children. They also need support to develop their own style of parenting free from any negative modelling that they have internalized from the past and also free from simply adopting the style of the children's mother. The therapist is thus called upon to use a supportive and didactic approach to foster the man's development as a father in a manner consistent with his self-awareness and growth as an individual. It is important to remember that we are dealing with a transitional generation of men who have typically lacked models for an active father role.

Larry's statement that "you don't win medals at the office" for being active with your children calls attention to another fact that significantly influences why many men today are diverted from being more involved as parents. There is little support in the work world or in the social lives of men for making parenting a primary part of their lives. One friend related a story of almost having been blackballed at the law firm where he was clerking because he had wanted to delay his bar exam if his first child was born right before the exam. Fortunately, a senior partner with a different attitude made known his support for being present around the time of birth and the situation was resolved. Men generally do not feel they can count on support in the workplace regarding parenting responsibilities. This is especially true for the more ordinary occurrences that require a parent's time, such as illness or school conferences, as well as for special events that are important for both child and parent to share.

Increasing father involvement in the lives of their children is made all the more important today because of the changing work patterns of women. Although mothers working outside the home become role models for a wider range of behaviors for women than was previously true and generally feel good about themselves, there is also less time available to the mother for the nurturing of children. Fathers becoming more involved in the nurturing end of home life is an essential response to this dilemma. For this to occur, however, change is needed for men on two levels: (1) there must be support on the social level from institutions, places of employment, and even peers; and (2) there must be educational or practical, along with emotional, support to learn how to fill a role that men have generally not been taught to fill.

Change on the social level will be difficult to achieve because it flies in the face of long-standing patterns that are based not only on gender stereotypes, but also on values that place economic concerns above familial ones. As a society we tend strongly to allow work concerns to dominate social ones, even to the point that we are blinded to the impact of unresolved personal problems on productivity for an individual.

Changing these values and priorities begins with doing what we can from our own positions of responsibility. As employers we can encourage or allow flexible time for both male and female employees to respond to the important needs of their children. In schools, day care programs, libraries, health care facilities, and so on, we can take into account the father role in our scheduling of events. The communications, and educational and supportive programming of these same institutions can reinforce the parenting role and responsibilities of the father. As individuals we can promote the active involvement of fathers through our simple recognition of men who are involved and through reaching out to them with ideas, encouragement, and support.

Therapists cannot change the social environment in which men must function. However, they can encourage and support men to not be passive in the face of social barriers to the changes that they are hoping to achieve. Many men, particularly those who never learned to question their own fathers' behaviors, have simply never considered asserting their needs to their bosses. Phil, in the previous chapter, was a prime example of a man who allowed himself to be pushed to the limits and believed that compliance was the manly option. With his therapist's exhortation, and some coaching and role playing, Phil was finally able to set some of his own limits on how much he would work. He was surprised at how readily his boss backed off when confronted with a decisive attitude. Not long after, Phil began to actively pursue a new job. The increased contact with one's children is sufficient reward for many men to limit work once the chronic pattern of overworking is identified and initially broken.

Therapists must recognize that men have generally lacked the social supports all their lives that would shape and prepare them for an active fathering role. Women typically have a flow of input about parenting issues that is integral to their functioning as mothers. Men do not often seek such input, but it is also not generally directed their way. To strengthen men's individual commitment to their role as fathers we need also to commit social resources that affirm the importance of this role and provide the relevant supports to confidently carry it out.

GROUP SUPPORT FOR FATHERS

One of the authors has been involved for the past 2 years in the efforts of a local Jewish Community Center to reach out to the fathers of toddlers. For several years previously the Center had created multiple activities for parents and their children, most of which were designed for mothers or attracted them almost exclusively. One group was specifically for fathers to bring a child for organized activities and projects. Mothers at the Center had always had ample opportunities for sharing and mutual support around their mothering concerns. Fathers had only the activity side covered, in part because it was expected that men would avoid any overt effort to promote sharing of parenting experiences.

To build a foundation for fathers that would address what it means to be a father with other men, a male psychologist (one of the authors) was hired as a co-facilitator for the group. While one facilitator was orchestrating craft projects, sing-a-longs, or parent–

child play, the psychologist was free to get to know the fathers on a personal level and explore with them their experiences and concerns as fathers.

When the group first began, the unstated model was the kind of group sharing that mothers did in similar settings. If the men could reach this point, the group would be a marked success. This goal did not take into account that the fathers in this group had little time during the week for one-to-one contact with their child and thus felt cheated when the focus turned away from the kids to each other. It was also a goal that did not give enough recognition to how aversive many men find structured group sharing of feelings and experiences. Moreover, it ignored that men may be able to talk about such concerns in their own way, instead of a way that is familiar to women.

After several weeks of having group discussions fizzle out, it was decided to stop trying to parallel the mothers' group approach and go with any ways that worked for the men. Once this shift occurred, the group took off. The male facilitator dropped efforts to draw the men into group sharing and simply roamed the playroom, engaging men in informal conversation about their children and how they felt about their role as fathers. When allowed to get to know the male facilitator on a one-to-one basis, the men began to open up. Initially they primarily responded to direct questions; in time they came up with their own questions. There was also a shift from maintaining a dialogue with the facilitator alone, to conversing with each other in one-to-one contact and groups of two or three.

Without the pressure to talk about feelings and concerns in a way that felt unnatural to the men and with the opportunity to build trust through a more gradual, personal, one-to-one process, men became able to discuss issues that earlier seemed only to elicit irritation or icy disinterest. It took only a matter of weeks after this shift in approach for the men to begin initiating a wide range of topics: from questions about how to deal with bed-wetting, potty-training, and sleep problems to their own feelings about being fathers, worries about the arrival of a second child, and frustration in competing with their wives for an equal say in child-rearing. One benchmark of success occurred on the day that one of the more reserved fathers came up to the facilitator with an oversized grin to report: "I met a friend at a fast food restaurant who, sure enough, asked me if I was babysitting for the kids. I told him, 'No way, I'm doing my thing as a father.' And, you know, it actually felt good to say that."

Another father who had to miss a session asked his wife to stop in and ask a question about their handling of a particular behavior of their son's. Some fathers who had to miss sessions sent their children with grandparents and even an uncle. Their sense of commitment to their children and to learning how to be the best fathers they could be came through loud and clear.

Until this class most of the men in the group seemed to have learned about how to be a parent primarily from their wives. As a result, they tended to feel less knowledgeable and less confident than their wives, which reinforced the carrying out of a subordinate role. Unfortunately, wives may inadvertently play into this attitude by holding on to their dominant role at home. It seemed like almost a relief to the fathers in the group to have a male figure who would discuss parenting issues with them and who supported their efforts at defining the kind of fathers they wanted to be. They also benefited tremendously by the opportunity for validation and support from other fathers, even though much of it was indirect. When the initial 10-week session ended and a new one began, some of the veterans who continued could be found talking with the newcomers with excitement about father issues and not just sports.

It was clear that by creating an environment and set of expectations that fit with how men deal with personal and affective issues, the capacity of men to share on this level could be brought out considerably. Although men may be most receptive to such an intervention when their children are young, creative efforts to support the father role with children of all ages—even older fathers with their adult children—are badly needed.

CONCLUSION

Our efforts in therapy with men have shown us that most men care very deeply about their children and want to be good fathers. They are often the last ones, however, to realize the ways that they may be shortchanging their children. When men are engaged in therapy, either for themselves or (ostensibly) for troubled children, they may well be motivated to learn about themselves and their role as fathers. When men are helped to explore their own father's shortcomings in an effort to understand themselves, they also have an opportunity to reassess how they are raising their own children. Their desire to not repeat the mistakes of their own fathers is commonly voiced and is usually a more palatable rationale for self-exploration than therapeutic talk about the need for expressing feelings and being open.

Often men have not known there were other ways to be a parent than the example set by their own fathers, and typically they have not believed they could talk about such things with others. Therapy is certainly one place that can and must validate this focus and help set the role of father in a broader context for male clients.

GUIDELINES

1. Men often are genuinely ignorant about the importance and impact of their role as fathers. They may well have never been asked in a constructive, nonthreatening way to examine themselves in this role. When approached from the vantage point that they do care and they may not have been aware of their deficiencies, many are surprisingly open to learn and to change.

2. Men generally have lacked support to learn the skills of parenting. They need guidance and resources, not simply exhortations to be more involved. The anxiety that comes from inadequate support and knowledge must be overcome, and that requires supportive opportunities to learn.

3. It is frequently necessary to help men disconnect from the negative role modelling of their own fathers. This requires exploring their relationships with their fathers and the learning about male and parental behavior that took place in this context. Getting in touch with positive aspects of their fathers and the desire to integrate these into one's own parenting is an important dividend of this exploration.

4. Encouragement to imitate their wives' approach to parenting will not likely be well received by husbands. Just as men need to find their own way of expressing emotions and communicating, they need models of parenting that recognize their maleness and validate their own constructive forms of father involvement.

5. There is little institutional or societal support and validation for a strengthened father role. Men need prodding and support to assert their needs as fathers within otherwise indifferent social frameworks.

REFERENCES

Osherson, S. (1986). *Finding our fathers: The unfinished business of man-hood.* New York: The Free Press.

Rubin, L. (1983). *Intimate strangers: Men and women together.* New York: Harper & Row.

·13·

Changing the Nature of Friendships between Men

BARRY GORDON and ROBERT S. PASICK

THE PROBLEM

As we have seen in Chapter 5, men tend to lack the kind of intimacy in their friendships that women seem to have. Moreover, they do not generally have the kind of blood-brother bond with another male that our popular myths and media images would have us believe they do. Indeed, our cultural myths about male bonds were formed in an ancient era when such solidarity was required for survival and the good of society necessitated cooperative involvement from everyone (Hammond & Jablow, 1987). Solidarity among men ends up being a secondary concern, at best, for the individual man struggling to meet the demands of modern society. Friendship is a fragmentary piece of life for most men, relegated to the spare time left once work and home obligations are met.

Male friendship today focuses on companionship, loyalty (though not of an Olympian quality anymore), and fun. Men tend to reserve their most personal, intimate contact for their special relationships with women. Pogrebin (1987) even suggests that men marry for friendship. However, one of the significant, though seldom-addressed, residual effects of the social changes occurring for women is that they are increasingly both physically and socially unavailable for men (Sherrod, 1987). Thus, men cannot confidently look to women to fill the role of best and only friends the way they typically have in the past.

The male friendship that is characteristic for most men is not oriented toward the direct sharing of personal and emotional concerns. Men do not regard their male connections as requiring the discussion of feelings and private matters that women do in order to feel close to a friend and benefit from the friendship. This kind of "inferred intimacy," as Sherrod (1987) calls it, works well for men until major problems or crises rear their ugly heads. At such times, inferred intimacy becomes deferred or nonexistent intimacy as men find their male companions too uneasy with matters of the heart to be there for them. When female partners are not available or when they are the focus of the crisis itself, many men find themselves alone with their problems. At times such as these, when men are more prone or ready to pursue more emotional depth in their friendships with men, they find it difficult to identify other males who are similarly inclined.

The social conditioning of men, our institutional requirements for men, and even our routines of daily life work against the formation of intimate male-to-male friendship. Urbanization, bureaucratization, and social and geographical mobility all tend to foster instrumental and expedient relationships and induce social isolation (Hammond & Jablow, 1987). However, our myths about friendship, as Hammond and Jablow (1987) point out, express the desire for the fulfillment of a wish. Although it may only surface at times of obvious need, men do indeed long for close bonds. Unfortunately, the pattern of so many men relying almost exclusively on their female partners for the satisfaction of this longing leaves men in a trap. They have allowed their skills and comfort with male connections to wither. Yet, out of overdependence on a woman, unwillingness to risk vulnerability even in their female relationships, or the unavailability of a trusted female, they may be left without any form of intimate friendship at a time of greatest need.

The conditions described above, which lead men to be socially isolated in times of crisis, may lead them to psychotherapy for help just because they are suffering from their aloneness. Ironically, a path most men eschew as unmanly becomes their only way out of a predicament largely induced by their need to be so manly. Indeed, helping men reevaluate and alter their connections to other men can be one of the effective means by which they are aided through psychotherapy.

THE ROLE OF THERAPY

When men come for psychotherapy, whether in a state of crisis or less commonly for their own personal growth, the issue of friendship is often an important element. There are three main reasons for this importance: (1) social support is a key factor in helping people through crises and even for promoting a person's development; (2) examining the quality of one's friendships provides a concrete vehicle for understanding the consequences of avoiding intimate connection, typically a significant problem for men; and (3) working on improving friendships provides a forum for changing interpersonal interaction and building support that is usually less risky or less charged than in a love relationship. For men who are experiencing emotional crises generally and for men who need to work on their interpersonal relating, especially on an intimate level, it will be useful to focus on a man's friendship patterns as part of therapy. Regardless of the nature of the problem, there are few men for whom this will not be at least secondarily relevant.

To focus on friendship as part of a therapeutic agenda with men requires the establishment of a rationale. Although women generally are open to therapy being a holistic enterprise, men typically must be convinced of the relevance of each new item that is introduced. A major therapeutic task, then, becomes taking men through the steps that clarify why their pattern of relating to friends is significant.

There are three steps that, although applicable to a variety of issues in therapy, are particularly relevant with friendship:

1. Awareness must be created that there is indeed a lack of intimate connection in the man's life. Druck (1985) points out that men often do not even think about friendship as a central or important concern. Many men have filled their lives in such a way that they believe they have obviated the need for the close friends they once had. Therapy needs to affirm that what was once important, though perhaps many years ago, is still important to them, even for sound functional reasons.

2. It must be demonstrated that to lack intimate connections does make a difference and, therefore, should be a priority concern. Many men carry the outlook that to have a friend is nice, but to need a friend is regarded as adolescent or immature (Goldberg, 1976). Ex-

ploring the value of past friendships, the effect of not having such friendships in the present, and the impact of centering one's friendship attachments in love relationships with women all add perspective and highlight the importance of this issue.

3. Belief must be fostered that something can be done to enrich one's friendships in a way that does not seem to pose a risk to one's masculinity. It is difficult enough for men to allow themselves to be vulnerable with others let alone to overtly act like intimate contact in a friendship is actually important to them. After all, when we seek closer friendship, we risk being rejected. Moreover, we may be seen as unmanly for even needing the closeness enough to have to pursue it. Ironically, acknowledging the risk within therapy can be turned into a positive by framing the issue as a manly way to face a difficult hurdle.

Therapy itself can be a bridge to the kind of intimate connections from which men otherwise steer clear. The relationship with the therapist can provide the kind of experience of intimacy, especially when it is with a male therapist, that the man may have simply never experienced. The therapist can give validation for the willingness to risk being vulnerable and, hopefully, himself models vulnerable behavior that represents strength rather than weakness. From a positive experience of intimate friendship set in the context of therapy, men are frequently encouraged to try, and to feel more comfortable with, efforts at establishing closer bonds on their own.

Therapy can be a practical as well as experiential bridge for the development of a friendship. The therapist can be helpful in this process by exploring the nature of past and present relationships of the male client. Examining these relationships can help to identify potential models and actual people for new or improved friendships. In this context can be found the qualities of intimate attachment that the man values and may already have experienced in his life. Looking at childhood and young adult friendships, and relationships with siblings, children, parents, past bosses, or mentors all help to promote the awareness that meaningful attachments are possible and have a significant, integral role in the man's life.

Often the therapist must be creative about finding ways to support men taking action in an area of social functioning which may be foreign and uncomfortable. Making use of the cognitive and social skills with which a man already is comfortable can offer leverage to promote new behaviors. One male client was helped to see that he was missing the spontaneous, mutual support he had found with peers in graduate school; however, he had become fatalistic about ever having such support again. He did know how to plan for a job change and to use his social networks to accomplish this. The therapist made use of this known skill to develop an approach to seeking new friends to which the client could commit. Being an inventive social planner can be as important for the therapist in promoting changes in relating as efforts directed at introspection and self-awareness.

THE PROCESS OF THERAPY

Helping men become aware of the need for friendship and the possibilities for developing deeper ties is not a one-dimensional, linear process. The therapeutic process itself is not this way either, and thus much of what needs to be done to foster the needed awareness, attitude, and actions around friendship is integral to the larger process. Within this context we can identify three elements generally common to a therapeutic process that especially need to be applied to male friendship patterns, and then a fourth which is specifically related to action steps around developing friendships: (1) freeing men from the negative impact of dysfunctional father–son relationships; (2) examining other common male obstacles to intimate behavior; (3) teaching men what to do with the tender feelings they do experience; and (4) planning action steps to take men beyond the traditional male role constraints to intimate friendship.

The lament of John (in Chapter 11) about his father never coming to see him in a single athletic event is a poignant example of the kind of sad story that so many men tell in therapy about their unfulfilled relationships with their fathers. Pogrebin (1987) tells us of a study which revealed that while four of five college-age women counted their mothers among their best friends, *none* of the young men so considered their fathers.

Male interaction with others is obviously shaped by how intimacy was experienced in the entire family of origin. However, the most dysfunctional modelling most typically is associated with how fathers related to their sons. When Tom, also from Chapter 11, found that his only way to connect to his father was through going to work with him, he also began a pattern that ran through his adulthood of substituting work for intimate connection. Bly (1986) points out that men cannot achieve separation because they have not achieved bonding in the first place with their fathers. The result is that a sense of loss continues to plague men and to play out in their other relationships. The direct effects include not considering intimacy as a priority, not trusting it, fearing that the desire for it is unmanly, and yet longing for it.

When therapy focuses on a man's relationship with his father, it usually identifies the single most powerful example of an unfulfilled intimate connection and its consequences. Phillip offers one example. He was gay and yearned for a loving, friendship-based, lasting couple relationship, yet also feared and avoided getting close to another man. He could not understand the simultaneous intensity of both sets of feelings. A breakthrough occurred when he came to the realization that his father had created a virtual taboo regarding conversation on an intimate level. Securing his father's approval meant avoiding intimacy with him and thus made the relationship an unfulfilling one. Within 6 weeks of arriving at this understanding, Phillip formed his first meaningful connection with another gay man.

Stan's father was a political activist and never seemed to have time for Stan unless he could combine it with his political work. Stan found it demeaning to compete for his father's time, but his own relationships with men were always formed around activities that surpassed the relationships in importance. Even in his marriage, Stan felt and acted like he himself was of secondary importance, until he began to see the origins of this pattern. When he stopped taking himself for granted, he could begin to expect reciprocity from his own efforts at relating.

Taking a thorough history of a man's relationship with his father should come early in the therapeutic process (see Chapter 11) because it provides a framework for understanding so much in how a man lives his life, including his handling of intimate connections. The paternal history-taking should cover the quality of the interaction with father, especially at significant developmental junctures, father's attitudes about intimacy, and his own pattern of relating to others. The value of taking an individual through an odyssey of his paternal interactions is not only that it uncovers behaviors that may have been modelled by the man's father, but it also heightens the self-awareness that the man carries into his present relationships. For example, one man purposely began to accept dinner invitations from friends in order to detach from work and strengthen these bonds after realizing that his own father had no friends and worked all the time. Moreover, he had never felt valued by his father and consequently for years had not treated himself as though he deserved much of anything. Taking time off to be with friends was a statement to himself that he did matter.

Helping men to understand the nature of their relationships to their fathers, then, is often a step that frees them to relate differently to all significant others. This work also often fosters renewed efforts to strengthen father–son attachments and, thus, may provide the adult son with an important new intimate connection. Going through this process affords the therapist the opportunity to affirm that having close relationships has been an appropriate desire all along, regardless of what was experienced with one's own father in growing up.

Making the translation from what he learned about intimacy in growing up to how he relates to others as an adult invariably involves uncovering how a man avoids intimate interactions and covers over his needs for closeness. The earlier example of Tom was of someone who had to substitute work for the attachment that he really wanted with his father. As an adult Tom filled his life with working and had only one friend with whom he made time to socialize. Excessive involvement with work is a pervasive pattern among men. It offers an excuse for not sustaining relationships that is both socially acceptable and usually monetarily, if not intrinsically, rewarding. As a result, it is easy to avoid examining the impact of this behavior. Reviewing an individual's work pattern and how it fits with his personal goals can expose the cost of overworking. One client, who is an attorney, bemoaned the fact that while he had several close friends living in town he rarely saw them even for lunch, because his calendar was always filled with obligatory social events. Another client, who was a sales representative, made a return visit to the city from which he had recently moved. While there he contacted four different people he wanted to see, but only one was a friend and the others were business acquaintances that he thought would be upset if they heard he was in town and did not call. It takes an assertive posture by the therapist to help men realize such patterns are chosen and have a detrimental effect.

Perhaps the most dysfunctional way men tend to fill the void of close friendships is through addictive behavior. One author (Druck, 1985) humorously declared, "Short of having sex together, two men may do just about anything as long as there is beer present" (p. 100). Having beer buddies and socializing over cocktails and dinner drinks will feel like he is carrying on friendships. Examining what needs these friendships do and do not meet often reveals that they are merely ways to evade intimacy. For men who are chemically dependent, it is not until they are recovering that they realize that such relationships were actually devoid of meaningful contact.

In cases where drugs or alcohol are misused to ease social contact, the therapist must confront the consequences of this behavior to avoid a plateau in social as well as personal growth. In fact, the deterioration of friendships is a common symptom and direct result of alcohol or drug abuse. It is at times necessary to take the position in therapy that addictive behavior of any kind will prevent the hope of change, and, conversely, the prospect of improved, deepened friendships is one positive source of motivation to stop the dependency.

The obstacles that therapy must address are not always found in such concrete behaviors. Each man develops his own self-protective devices, e.g., humor, sarcasm, and defensiveness, often learned in the context of his early familial and paternal relationships. Such behaviors are not readily seen by the men as keeping people at a safe distance. The therapist can use the therapy context itself to demonstrate the consequences of these distancing ways of relating. One 40-year-old client, Leonard, did not realize until therapy how much he had been pained by his father's explosive and rejecting treatment. Through therapy he was able to then also see how as a result he had developed the persona of a boisterous, affable clown to draw people and attention to him in a way that felt safe. The therapist had to confront Leonard with how he carried out this persona even in the therapy sessions in order to help him face how entrenched it was. He explained to himself and his therapist with considerable remorse, "I was so into it and so good at it that even I never realized I was just wearing a mask. I know now that I desperately need to drop that mask, but I'm honestly afraid I can't do it. You're the only one who knows me without it besides my wife."

Thus, identifying the ways men create their own barriers to closeness is a requisite step in therapy to releasing the emotional energy they do have for relationships. Tracing the roots of these avoiding behaviors to their fathers and their family of origin makes them more understandable and amenable to change. However, the motivation for change may require linking the lack of closeness to the underlying sense of loneliness men often acknowledge once they feel secure enough in therapy.

Leonard faced a new dilemma once he became aware of how he kept others at a safe distance. He realized, as many men do in therapy, that he had a softer, even tender side, but he still did not know if he could get himself to express that side to others, especially males from whom he most expected rejection.

For many men the language to express intimacy is foreign. They not only feel uncomfortable, but may actually lack the ability to put into words what they feel. Some need help knowing they do have such feelings. They may need to be reminded of poignant events or reactions to certain songs or movies to heighten awareness so they can attach words to describe what they feel. It is critical that they be allowed to develop their own manner of expression at their own pace. It is one of the intrinsic rewards of therapy to experience men opening up who have spent their whole lives repressing feelings they could not entrust to others. The nonjudgmental support and validation men can get in therapy fosters the growth of this tender side. Of course, the disclosing itself acts as its own reward because the men inevitably feel more whole, relaxed, and at peace.

Getting men to extend this vulnerable behavior outside of therapy is a difficult challenge. Becoming more conscious of their loneliness does not of itself reduce the aversion to being vulnerable by seeking closer ties to others. This is especially true because it is not simply a self-defeating projection that they cannot expect receptiveness from most other males. Helping men to surmount the fear of exposing their new-found capacity for intimacy involves work in two directions. First, it is possible to broaden a man's own definition of what it means to be masculine. When football stars perform in ballets and changing stations for babies are placed in men's rooms, it signals that the public world is more prepared for men to act in ways beyond the male stereotypes. These small public steps can be used to support changes in men's private behaviors. Encouraging men to try new roles and ways of being themselves leads them to a wider self-acceptance and a freedom to consider a broader range of behaviors as no less masculine than the traditional ones. When their own experiences are affirming and rewarding, such as spending one-to-one time with a child, discussing their own childhood feelings, or allowing themselves to risk embarrassment in an activity such as learning to ice skate with a wife who acts as teacher, they begin to be less guarded about the reactions of others.

Secondly, to promote experiences that broaden a man's definition of masculinity often requires the man to get beyond the environmental constraints that impose their traditional roles. Pogrebin (1987) concluded that women who get to know men outside of traditional gender roles are more likely to be able to form friendships with them. Druck (1985) related a story about two men who met at a seminar without knowing each other's occupations and formed an instant friendship, only to discover later they were business competitors who had hated each other without ever having met. Work roles are a particularly strong barrier for men, as we have discussed elsewhere, not only because the work ethic is tied to competitive behavior, but also because work readily offers men a safe, manly subject to talk about that allows them to avoid intimacy. For men to locate other men who will be receptive to friendship on an intimate basis probably means looking to environments where traditional males do not dominate, and thus relate where they can to other men without the crutch of traditional roles.

Identifying concrete actions men can take in order to develop changed friendship patterns requires inventiveness and facing the degree of risk-taking in which men are willing to engage. One step for men is to consciously attempt to connect to others without using their work identity. This exercise pushes men not only to risk through dropping some of their usual ways of avoiding intimacy, but also forces them to explore themselves to find other dimensions they can present to others. It is jolting to men to realize how much they tend to rely on this traditional identity and how little else of themselves they stay in touch with.

Since men do spend so much of their time invested in work and since work provides a comfort zone in their social relating, the work environment may need to be used as a locus of change efforts for those who are unable to try new ways of relating outside of work. By suggesting that they make efforts to connect to work peers outside of their usual capacity, even to commit to taking time at lunch or on breaks to relate on a nonwork basis, helps men see that they do not have to be consumed by their traditional roles.

Another dimension of work that can open new channels of relating is the potential to find a mentor or become a mentor. The structure of male relationships to superiors or subordinates is typically narrow and restrictive, tied to corporate objectives, institutional demands, and codes of conduct. Men lack the kind of strong, cultural rituals that past generations and different cultures have used to validate bonds with parental substitutes. Bly (1986) stresses the importance for male development of a "male mother," someone whose "kindness, savvy, spiritual energy, . . . psychic knowledge" (p. 47) serve to guide and welcome the young male into the larger society and his adult, male responsibilities. The mentor role, whether one is the guide or the follower, offers a way to integrate the functional side of masculinity with the relational side. Being a mentor or having a mentor provides a vehicle for the expression or receipt of nurturing and growth-inducing behaviors. Such ties already exist on a functional level for many men, but operate by the rules of inferred, rather than directly expressed intimacy that men honor. These relationships, with a little effort and risk, can become fruitful sources of deeper bonds.

Just as the mentor relationship can be a bridge to intimate connection, father–child interactions—the prototype of the mentor—can provide fertile territory to risk expression of one's tender side. Encouraging men to test the preconceived limits of their relationships to their own aging parents or to alter the emotional neutrality they may have conveyed to their own children gives men the opportunity to discover their own dormant desire for meaningful attachments. These familial ties, including efforts with siblings, are extremely helpful in opening up men's views of the value of friendship. When efforts to strengthen these family bonds work, as they so often do at least partially, they help break down the belief that relationships cannot operate on an intimate level. When efforts fail, they still serve to demonstrate the deep need that men have for such relationships, even when they must be substitutes for the primary ones that have been unrequited.

Becoming a father for the first time opens up tender, loving feelings that men may well have not believed possible. On the feeling level, the period in a man's life when he has young children can be a wonderful opportunity to experience his desire for intimate attachment. However, the way men approach their new fatherhood role can lead them to fix all their emotions in the bond with the new child, as though sharing themselves with others will dilute their loyalty and responsibilities as father. Moreover, with the usual male commitment to work added to the requirements as a parent (and spouse of a new parent), men are left with little time to maintain even superficial friendships. Men in a support group for new fathers, co-led by one of the authors, identified the area of keeping friends as one of their primary concerns. These men seemed to believe that their placing friendship on hold while their children were infants would be a temporary casualty of new fatherhood. The reality for most men is that friendships continue to be on hold, since the tide of male obligatory behavior does not recede on its own.

As critical as it is to help men give expression to intimate feelings, these efforts are relatively futile if one does not succeed in getting them to make room in their lives to put this into practice. Having new fathers retain a night out or other regular social connection with friends is one type of action that makes use of the opportunity posed by an emotion-laden new phase of life. Securing commitments to set limits on the work day, to emphasize group instead of loner activities, and to set up lunch appointments for purely social motives are ways to establish that a man must include friendship-building on his personal agenda and decide to make it a priority.

One male client who had become isolated by work and a stagnant marriage chose to volunteer at a hunger center. His goal was not to meet people and make friends, but rather to get in touch with a lost sense of his capacity to give to others. Taking action on this goal of giving expression to a side of himself he had valued and placing himself in an environment where he could do so did far more than remind him he could be altruistic: "It taught me that I could open up and risk with others, when I'd long given up on ever doing so again. Even if no one at the center wanted me as a friend, I knew I could really be there the next time an opportunity presented itself." Making the commitment is the turning point in therapy, not just discovering that the feelings are there.

The transition from a man becoming aware of how he has placed himself in a state of isolation and loneliness to committing to change involves an interim stage of strengthening his sense of self. The man who volunteered at the hunger center could not make this choice until he had explored the kind of person he really wanted and needed to be. Men spend years constructing an image of the kind of man their fathers and mothers want them to be and to whom their possible future mates will be attracted. When they come to terms with how much they have feared making their own choices and developing their own masculine and total identity, they are better prepared to risk exposing their true selves to the test of intimate friendship. When they arrive at this point, being challenged to extend themselves with others offers a vital and meaningful vehicle for self-actualization.

A MEN'S GROUP

For some men, committing to deeper relationships necessitates the kind of emotional greenhouse a men's group can provide. The experience of one of the authors in conducting such a group follows.

The therapist formed the group by asking several male clients to attend an introductory meeting on a Saturday morning. He explained the initial session was exploratory, and required no commitment to the following six sessions.

The therapist opened the first meeting by discussing his hope that the group would help each member improve his relationships with spouses, children, families, and friends. To accomplish this, he said, the group must provide a supportive anad safe atmosphere where men could discuss their concerns. The therapist also hoped the participants would realize their problems were not unusual, learn they could accept and provide support for other men, improve their listening skills, and increase their awareness of the common pressures they face as men in our society. Overall, the therapist hoped each member would come to value the support and friendship of the other men.

First Session

Nine of the eleven men invited came to the first meeting, which was initially filled with apprehension from the participants and the group leader. Coffee and donuts were provided to allow the group to informally chat before getting to business. After the leader expressed the above goals for the group, they followed this agenda:

1. The men introduced themselves and disclosed what had prompted them to enter therapy. They were asked to not reveal their professions.

2. The therapist led several brainstorming exercises, which focused on the socialization they received as American males, their reactions to key terms ("mother," "father," "friend," "woman," etc.), and their feelings about being in the group. This approach allowed the group to get comfortable.
3. The group discussed the importance of confidentiality.
4. The group agreed upon a time for future meetings.

Each subsequent meeting followed the same general format, which included:

• The initial "schmoozing" over coffee and donuts. This unstructured time permitted the members to discuss whatever they wanted. The most popular topics were sports, politics, and current events. During this time, friendships began to develop.
• A "go-round" where each man talked briefly about the developments in his life. These usually focused on work or family issues. Feedback was encouraged.
• A structured input from the group leader, including some brief remarks about the topic of the day, listed below. These were often personal and light. This preceded a group exercise that required each man to write personal responses to the day's topic. Members would share their reactions, then discuss the group's findings.
• The remaining time provided the opportunity to discuss more thoroughly whatever issues were the most provocative. At first, few dared take advantage of this time, but this pattern changed by the third or fourth session. The daily topics the group explored are listed below.

Second Session: Men and Work

Each member discussed how he felt about his work situation.
The notion that men are "raised to work."
Comfort at work relative to comfort at home.
Work-related stress.

Third Session: Men as Husbands

The relationships of men and the significant women in their lives (including mothers, wives, sisters, and daughters).

What would men like to better understand about women?
Gender differences in the "definitions of self."

Fourth Session: Men as Fathers

Men's relationships with their fathers.
Concept of "father hunger."
Men's relationships with their children.

Fifth Session: Men and Friendships

Men's relationships with other men.
Obstacles to friendship between men, including homophobia.
Best friends: then and now.
Friendship and the men's group.

Sixth and Seventh Sessions: Family of Origin

Genograms.
Sculpting the family meal time.
Sibling relationships.

After completing the seven-session program, all the participants were sufficiently enthusiastic to continue meeting. The format remained the same, although the topics came more often from the members than the group leader. These included controlling tempers, parental influence, emotions, sex, balancing careers and families, divorce, having fun as an adult, and understanding women. Some of these subjects were covered in one or two sessions; others, such as family of origin, spanned several weeks. With each meeting more time was devoted to the go-rounds, where each man would talk about his personal life.

The group's guidelines were designed to create a safe, noncompetitive atmosphere where men could talk openly about themselves and their problems. It was not a confrontational group. The men listened to each other but delivered feedback very carefully, and avoided unnecessarily negative and critical remarks. This tone initially surprised the group, but in a later discussion they realized it was their manner of respecting the other, which was not their style in other settings. They made genuine efforts to listen and be supportive.

Initially, the men were reluctant to present specific or current problems to the group. They would often skip a session during a personal crisis, and not discuss it until it had been resolved. Gradually, they trusted the group to not scorn or reject them if they admitted they needed help with a problem. Many felt acknowledging their pain was the most difficult aspect of group therapy.

Sometimes the men's reluctance to confront a fellow member went to extremes. One participant announced that he planned to leave town and his girlfriend for a new job. Only after the man had left the meeting did the others express their disagreement with the decision. They explained they did not feel justified giving him direct critical feedback. After discussing this incident, however, they grew more willing to speak their minds.

Another positive result of the group sessions was a growing awareness of what it takes for men to make changes. For example, after one man changed jobs, the others stated they knew 6 months before that he hated his job and should leave it. They realized, however, that he would not make the move until he recognized its importance, and all their advice could not accelerate the process.

Eighteen months after the group's first session several members agreed to be interviewed about their experience for a therapists' conference. All agreed they had benefited significantly from the process. This is reflected in their comments:

> "I thought I was a cripple to have to go to therapy. The group made me feel I was not bizarre, nor alone with my problems."

> "Through the group I learned the benefits of listening. You don't have to solve people's problems. It helps just to listen."

> "I learned to respect others when they are hurting."

> "I realized you don't always have to be right."

> "I overcame my fear of being judged by other men."

> "This helped me tremendously with my relationship with my daughter. The other men told me I didn't have to be so critical."

> "I felt validated as a man."

> "I felt I was not alone. Though I never have, I knew I could call any member of the group if I needed help."

> "It gave me a greater appreciation of men—how they think, how they feel, how they struggle."

Such experiences have led us to believe men's support groups can be an integral component in helping men change. A particularly important benefit of the group is helping men sustain and strengthen changes by relying on the support of other men. Many men in the group discussed here continued in the group long after their individual or family therapy had ended. The group enabled them to continue to focus on important issues in their lives, in a setting where they could feel comfortable being vulnerable and intimate with other men.

GUIDELINES FOR HELPING MEN DEEPEN FRIENDSHIPS

1. If the therapy relationship itself feels like a friendship, i.e., it operates on an intimate, caring level, it will serve as a model and promote the seeking of this quality of friendship elsewhere.

2. Identifying actual intimate bonds from a man's past, especially when compared with loneliness and friendship voids in the present, will be a motivating force for change because it makes concrete what the man is missing.

3. It must be recognized that it is not easy and will take time to reverse the pattern of keeping friendships superficial and secondary. Small risks and a willingness to persist must be supported.

4. Utilize familiar concepts that a man can readily relate to, such as the idea of applying networking or strategic planning—common work-related practices—to developing friendships.

5. Encourage men to consider potential friendship ties with other men on a broad and nontraditional basis. However, do not denigrate traditional paths to friendship, such as sports or work, since the problem is not how men find the connection, but how they relate once they have made it.

6. Support whatever openness in relating is accessible in the man, rather than criticizing the lack of it. Sometimes creative reframing is required to expose a hidden desire and capacity for intimate relating that can be built upon.

REFERENCES

Bly, R. (1986, April/May). Men's initiation rites. *Utne Reader*, pp. 42–49.

Druck, K. (1985). *The secrets men keep.* New York: Ballantine Books.

Index